CREATING BEAUTIFUL, CONFIDENT

smiles

DR. MARTY VERBIC

CREATING BEAUTIFUL, CONFIDENT smiles

A SMART PATIENT'S GUIDE TO CHOOSING AN ORTHODONTIST

SPECIAL SECTION ON INVISALIGN

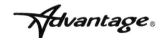

Published by Advantage, Charleston, South Carolina.
Member of Advantage Media Group.

ADVANTAGE is a registered trademark, and the Advantage colophon is a trademark of Advantage Media Group, Inc.

Printed in the United States of America.

10 9 8 7 6 5 4 3 2 1

ISBN: 978-1-59932-891-1
LCCN: 2018942083

Book design by Megan Elger.

This publication is designed to provide accurate and authoritative information in regard to the subject matter covered. It is sold with the understanding that the publisher is not engaged in rendering legal, accounting, or other professional services. If legal advice or other expert assistance is required, the services of a competent professional person should be sought.

Advantage Media Group is proud to be a part of the Tree Neutral® program. Tree Neutral offsets the number of trees consumed in the production and printing of this book by taking proactive steps such as planting trees in direct proportion to the number of trees used to print books. To learn more about Tree Neutral, please visit **www.treeneutral.com**.

Advantage Media Group is a publisher of business, self-improvement, and professional development books and online learning. We help entrepreneurs, business leaders, and professionals share their Stories, Passion, and Knowledge to help others Learn & Grow. Do you have a manuscript or book idea that you would like us to consider for publishing? Please visit **advantagefamily.com** or call **1.866.775.1696**.

To Wanda:

You remind me every day about the higher purpose of my life and work.

table of contents

acknowledgments

I'd like thank my staff for finding all of the photos and patient stories contained in this book and for making it possible for us to help as many people as we can to achieve healthy, confident smiles.

Thank you to all of the orthodontists and business leaders from whom I have accumulated the sum of my knowledge. I would not have become the leader I am today without your wisdom and coaching.

Thank you to the people of Advantage|ForbesBooks for helping with the organization and publishing of this book.

introduction

I became an orthodontist by taking a road less traveled. Chemical engineering had been my dream since taking my first chemistry class in high school. I went to college and became an engineer, started working in the field, and quickly found out it wasn't for me. I didn't have a passion for it. I was stuck inside an oil refinery, on call around the clock and on weekends and holidays. My only human interaction was with four other engineers and we had minimal contact with the outside world. I felt disconnected from people and it was difficult to feel like I was making any real difference. I shared my feelings with family and friends and started to think about new potential career paths.

At the time, my mom was working in an insurance office located next to an orthodontic practice. One day, she was sharing my feelings of professional discontent with the orthodontist and he immediately said, "Well, I *love* my job. Tell Marty to stop by and see what orthodontics is all about. He'll see why I love my job. And maybe it'll be for him too."

So, I did. I spent a day following Dr. Stanciu around while he examined and treated patients and interacted with his staff, parents of patients, and children. I saw teenagers who were so happy to get their braces off they couldn't stop grinning. I saw tears of joy, tons of smiles, very happy parents, and balloons. It was incredible. I loved it and thought, what a great profession.

I immediately realized this was a career where I could make a profound difference in peoples' lives. By combining my engineering mind with dental schooling, I could learn to fix teeth and create beautiful smiles for children and adults. So, I went for it; I couldn't turn away from an opportunity to work in a field where I could interact daily with lots of people and see real, positive results day in and day out. I took the dental school entrance exam and was accepted to the University of Illinois at Chicago, College of Dentistry. After dental school, I completed a three-year residency program at the University of Illinois at Chicago and earned a specialty certificate in orthodontics and an MS degree in oral science. The dental school and orthodontic residency years went by in a flash because I loved what I was learning. About six months after finishing my residency, I met a doctor who was retiring after a forty-two-year career and wanted to sell his practice to another orthodontist to keep it going. And that is how Verbic Orthodontics was born.

SO WHY AM I WRITING THIS BOOK?

New patients walk into my practice every day. Most of the time, they are not smiling, their shoulders are slumped and they are often shy. We take initial photos before starting treatment, and many of the patients—children and adults—won't smile in these photos because they are embarrassed about their teeth. It's truly heartbreaking. Yet, within only about six months of treatment, there is a noticeable difference in my patients. They start to smile, become more talkative, and stand taller. They talk about socializing more at school, raising their hand in class, and about going to dances and parties. I see their confidence improving right before my eyes. Orthodontic treatment changes them. Patients often don't realize how the process can change them and the entire trajectory of their lives.

Creating beautiful, confident smiles for as many people as possible is my passion. But because it is my passion, I sometimes forget that not everyone shares my obsession with all-things-teeth. I wrote this book to answer questions, the many questions that I get every day from my patients and the parents of my patients. I want to answer these questions not only for my actual and potential patients, but also for everyone out there who is considering orthodontic treatment for themselves or for their child.

Some of my patients' questions are based on misconceptions or preconceived notions of treatment. In my desire to reassure them, I've spent a lot of time thinking about how best to explain orthodontic treatment. This book dispels many misconceptions that are floating around about orthodontics and answers many of the common questions I hear every week such as:

"Why do so many people have crowded teeth?"

"Why does my eight-year-old child need braces?"

"How can I pay for treatment?"

"Will I need to have teeth pulled?"

"What if I really can't afford treatment for my child?"

This book takes the mystery out of orthodontic treatment for anyone considering it for themselves or their child. Since orthodontic treatment is a big investment, finding a top-quality orthodontic practice to partner with is important. After reading this book, you will be prepared to ask important questions that will guide you in finding the best orthodontic practice for you or your child.

Personally, I learn a lot more when I read something versus listening to something. So, I thought there might be more visual learners like me out there, and that writing a book like this would be a helpful tool to have when researching options for orthodontic treatment. When you go to an orthodontist's office, it is often busy and hectic and you might hear the answers to your questions, but because you are distracted, it may go in one ear and out the other. This book is my answer to this potential problem. You can read this book in the quiet of your home or office or even on vacation and have time to process and understand the information.

I also hope this book can take the fear out of financing orthodontic treatment, and encourage reluctant patients to take the first step by calling and scheduling an orthodontic consultation. When parents realize their child has crooked or crowded teeth, their first thought is, "Oh, no! How will we pay for braces?" They automatically think they will never be able to afford treatment. But this is no longer the case. There are so many great financing options, orthodontic insurances, HSAs, and FSAs available today. And, for those who really cannot afford treatment, there are wonderful charity organizations that provide treatment practically free of charge to those who qualify. In fact, my office works with charities like Smiles Change Lives and Donated Orthodontic Services. Their mission is to donate orthodontic treatment at little to no cost to children in financial need. Verbic Orthodontics is honored to partner with these programs.

Orthodontic treatment really isn't as expensive, time consuming, or painful as people think. New technology is constantly being developed, standards of practice have changed significantly, and costs have decreased dramatically. All of this means that getting treatment for orthodontic problems today is *very* different from what it used to be. Orthodontists are here to help and we really do have a passion for making a difference in peoples' smiles ... and their lives.

chapter one

THE SCIENCE BEHIND CROOKED, CROWDED, AND MISSING TEETH

It happens all the time. A dad comes in with his child for an orthodontic consult and says, "How did my child's teeth get so crooked when my teeth and my wife's teeth are perfectly straight? It must be my wife's genetics!" Then, at the next appointment, the mom brings the child and asks the same question and says, "It must be my husband's genetics!" It's actually quite funny to watch it play out. Dad blames Mom; Mom blames Dad. I laugh and tell them that, most of the time, it's really no one's fault. Crooked, crowded, and missing teeth usually just happen.

—DR. VERBIC

GENETICS

So, why *are* some people's teeth so crowded; why *do* some people develop a big overbite? One of the first things I like to say to my patients is, "This isn't your fault. There really isn't anything you could have done to prevent it, and it's mostly hereditary." There are many orthodontic conditions that are almost always partly due to genetics. These include issues with jaw size or asymmetry, tooth size and shape, missing teeth, extra teeth, teeth that come in sideways, crowded teeth, cleft lips and palates, deep bites, keeping baby teeth too long, and not getting adult teeth in on time. These conditions may occur due to the genetics within a family, and it's possible the genetics skipped a generation or two. So, the orthodontic issues present in your teeth or your child's teeth might be great-grandpa's fault.

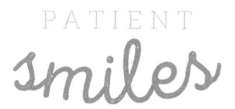
PATIENT *smiles*

Our adopted daughter was born with a cleft lip and palate. Genetics are so complicated; we know it is not anyone's fault that she was born with this disorder. We just knew from the beginning that we would work tirelessly with her doctor, surgeon, and Dr. Verbic to correct the jaw and orthodontic issues that she had already and would face as she grew older. After several surgeries to work on fixing the cleft palate, our daughter was in phase 1 braces by age eight to address a severe underbite. Dr. Verbic was so lovely to work with; he was so encouraging to our daughter throughout the whole process. Now, at thirteen years old, our daughter still needs quite a bit of work, including either another jaw surgery or a special procedure to realign the plates in her palate, another round of braces and possibly some cosmetic work. Yes, this has certainly been a challenging process and our daughter is still very self-conscious of her teeth, but she is a trooper and she has developed perseverance in the face of this challenge. We are so thankful for her great team of doctors, including Dr. Verbic, who continue to help her and us face this disorder head on. One day, our daughter will have a beautiful, healthy smile and all of this struggle will have been worth it. —HELEN M.

EVOLUTIONARY FACTORS

In addition to genetics passed down from generation to generation, there is an overarching, evolutionary reason that plays a role in the crowding of teeth.[1] This evolutionary reason helps explain why humans in general have crowded teeth or large overbites. Looking at it from our perspective, if crowded teeth are harder to clean and cause the development of gum disease more frequently than straight teeth do, then why would so many people's teeth come in crowded when there is no evolutionary advantage to them doing so?

Weston Price, a dentist practicing in the 1920s, wanted answers to this question. He set out to find the answers by studying indigenous people from Africa, Australia, the Polynesian Islands, and Northern Canada. One of his observations was that none of these indigenous people had crooked teeth or large overbites. Their teeth were perfectly straight and their jaws were well formed.[2]

This led to another question. If indigenous people of the world do not have orthodontic problems, then why do people in developed parts of the world have them? One theory is that the jaw bones of people who live in the developed world have shrunk over time because of the softer, processed foods they eat, compared to the diets of indigenous people. The human body does not want to expend energy to maintain unnecessarily large jaw bones when the diet is softer. This

---

1   Weston A. Price, *Nutrition and Physical Degeneration: A Comparison of Primitive and Modern Diets and Their Effects* (New York: Medical Book Department of Harper & Brothers, 1939).

2   Ibid.

is a well-documented, evolutionary adaptation that helps humans survive by reducing the number of calories they must consume.[3]

A similar adaptation can be seen in people who have been paralyzed from the waist down. Their leg muscles and bones shrink, and the leg bones become less dense. This is because the body has adapted to not expend energy on parts of the body that are not in use.[4] In effect, the body asks itself, "Why waste energy to support something that you're not using?" Therefore, if modern humans are eating softer diets that don't require strong jaw muscles and jaw bones to eat, then the jaws are going to shrink in size.

In his studies, Price observed that the children of Australian aborigines who moved into major population centers of Australia and ate modern diets developed crowded teeth and smaller jaws over a short time. In fact, the changes in jaw structure happened within one generation.

You might think the teeth themselves would also try to shrink in shape and size to fit the smaller jaws, so they would not become crowded. Good thinking, but instead, more people in the developed parts of the world are *missing* teeth. The body is adapting to smaller jaw sizes by reducing not the *size* of the teeth but the *number* of teeth in the jaws. More and more people are missing wisdom teeth. More and more people are missing premolar teeth. Some people are even missing incisors, which are the front teeth. People who are missing wisdom teeth should feel fortunate because wisdom teeth

---

3   Ibid.; T. P. Stein and C. E. Wade, "Metabolic Consequences of Muscle Disuse Atrophy," *J Nutr.* 135 (suppl 7, 2005): 1824S–1828S; Gerard Karsenty, "Convergence Between Bone and Energy Homeostases: Leptin Regulartion of Bone Mass, *Cell Metabolism* 4, no. 5 (November 2006): 341-348, www.sciencedirect.com/science/article/pii/S1550413106003378

4   L Giangregorio and CJ Blimkie, "Skeletal adaptations to alterations in weight-bearing activity: a comparison of models of disuse osteoporosis," *Sports Med* 32, no. 7 (2002): 459–476, https://www.ncbi.nlm.nih.gov/pubmed/12015807

often become impacted and need to be removed by an oral surgeon. Missing these particular teeth is actually a really good thing.

As part of their orthodontic treatment, patients missing premolar and incisor teeth frequently need bridges or implants to replace them or for the spaces to be closed. These people (or parents) are sometimes upset they need to bear the additional burden of having teeth replaced.

> One mother got nervous that her daughter would need to have her missing premolars replaced. I shared that this is more common than she'd think, and then, to calm her daughter in the dental chair, I smiled and said, "On the plus side, you are more evolutionarily advanced than people who have all of their teeth." They thought it was great.
>
> **—DR. VERBIC**

After reading this, it may seem like there is little we can do as parents to prevent our children from needing braces, and for the most part, this is true. Most causes of crooked or crowded teeth, bad bites and missing teeth are genetic and/or evolutionary in nature. But, beyond genetic and evolutionary factors, there are several behavioral factors that might play a role in the development of orthodontic problems.[5]

BEHAVIORAL FACTORS

Behavioral factors may play a role in orthodontic problems, including bad habits, injury, and dental disease.

---

5   Parag Deshmukh, "Hereditary Factors Etiology of Malocclusion," *SlideShare*, accessed at www.slideshare.net/pdeshmukh1/hereditary-factors-etiology-of-malocclusion

BAD HABITS

Bad habits are hard to break for us and for our children. Habits in children can play a role in the development of orthodontic issues, including thumb or finger sucking, tongue thrusting, lip sucking/biting, nail biting, abnormal swallowing, mouth breathing, and even poor posture. Helping our children kick these habits and seeking medical or dental evaluation if swallowing, breathing, or posture problems are noticed is vital in preventing orthodontic problems.

INJURY

Injury is another factor that may lead to orthodontic problems. Of course, in the majority of cases, there is not much you can do as a parent to prevent accidents, and any resulting tooth or jaw injury, from happening. However, insisting that your children wear helmets while biking, skiing, skateboarding, and playing football and using mouth guards when playing contact sports is essential for safety.

DENTAL DISEASE

However, the biggest behavioral factor contributing to orthodontic problems, is dental disease, which can lead to early loss of baby teeth. Baby teeth act as space maintainers for the adult teeth that will eventually come into the mouth to replace them. When baby teeth are lost early, the adult teeth that replace them usually don't come in straight. This is because the teeth beside that baby tooth shifts into the empty space if the baby tooth is lost early. This blocks the adult tooth that is supposed to come in, and ultimately disrupts the positioning. Most baby teeth that are lost early are due to infections caused by cavities that get so large they cannot be repaired with fillings by a dentist. The dentist sometimes has no choice but to remove the baby tooth to prevent the infection from spreading to the jaws and the rest of the body. When the baby tooth is removed, the dentist should place a space maintainer to prevent the surrounding teeth from encroaching upon the space. This will give the adult tooth that comes in the best possible chance of coming in straight. So, as parents, it is important to help our children choose healthy foods that are low in sugar and high in nutrients, and to help our children brush their teeth at least twice a day, develop good flossing habits, and use a fluoride rinse, in some cases. Good nutrition and good oral hygiene will help prevent cavities, tooth infections, and the eventual orthodontic problems that they could create through early loss of baby teeth.

So, as you can see, there are many factors involved in the science behind crooked, crowded, and missing teeth. In *most* cases, there is nothing you could have done to prevent the problems from developing. In *some* cases, though, there are things you can do to prevent and/or slow the progression of problems.

In addition to breaking bad habits, preventing injury, and preventing dental disease, another important thing you can do is take your child to the orthodontist by age seven for an early orthodontic evaluation.

chapter two

THE IMPORTANCE OF EARLY ORTHODONTIC EVALUATION

> *I had a new patient a few weeks ago who had been referred to me by her family dentist. She was young, only seven years old, so my first interaction was with her mom. After we greeted each other, the child's mom blurted out, "She is only seven years old! Why did our dentist refer her for an evaluation at seven? This seems way too young. She's only lost four baby teeth so far. I only got braces when I was fifteen—after I had lost all of my baby teeth. Please explain to me the reason for this evaluation."*
>
> **—DR. VERBIC**

I hear reactions and questions like this quite a bit when I explain the importance of an orthodontic consult by the time a child is seven years old. I always respond with a version of the following: "You'd be surprised by all the problems I see in teenagers we could have helped prevent from happening if they had just visited me a few years prior.

I could have saved them from needing invasive surgery and I could have saved them thousands of dollars."

Timing is everything when it comes to orthodontic treatment in children. Seven years old seems young, and to be fair, it is very different advice compared to what was given just a decade or so ago. The timeline for orthodontic evaluation used to be scheduled for when all the baby teeth were gone and all of the adult teeth were in. But the field of orthodontics has changed dramatically based on new research and treatment options.

RECOGNITION OF ORTHODONTIC PROBLEMS THAT CAN BE TREATED EARLY

Many orthodontic problems that can be corrected easily during childhood cannot be corrected without more-invasive treatment, such as surgery, if the problems are left untreated past puberty and into adulthood. This is because when the jaw bones are still growing, orthodontists have some ability to control the magnitude and direction of their growth. After most growth has stopped, following puberty, patients with abnormal jaw growth may be left only with the choice of surgical correction or compromised results. The American Association of Orthodontists (AAO) recommends children have an orthodontic evaluation at the age of seven.[6] This is because at age seven it is possible to both determine if there are any abnormalities in jaw growth and it is possible to intervene with orthopedic correction, if needed. The AAO also provides a list of the common orthodontic problems in younger children that require orthodontic referral and potential phase 1 treatment. The following listed problems are illustrated in Figure 2.1. It also lists other issues to look for in your child,

---

6   "Frequently Asked Questions," American Association of Orthodontists, www. aaoinfo.org/frequently-asked-questions

including speech difficulties, thumb sucking, mouth breathing, and so on, which indicate that an evaluation by an orthodontist is important:

- Anterior Crossbite

- Posterior Crossbite

- Crowding

- Open bite

- Protrusion

- Deep bite

- Underbite

- Spacing Issues

Anna K. was referred to me by her family dentist because her top canine tooth had fallen out at age thirty. At her first appointment, we used special x-ray techniques to find out what was going on. It turned out Anna had an impacted adult top canine tooth; the tooth that had fallen out was a baby tooth. And we saw she also had an impacted adult tooth on the bottom. So, the only treatment plan available was to pull the other baby tooth and perform a minor surgery to place two special bands within the gum on the impacted adult teeth to help pull them into the mouth. The patient also needed braces for quite a while. If this patient had been evaluated by an orthodontist when she was eight years old, the fact that her adult teeth were moving in the wrong direction would have been seen right away and treatment could have been started. If the baby teeth had been pulled earlier, there would have been much better odds that the teeth would have come in straight on their own.

—DR. VERBIC

Problems to Watch
for in Seven Year Olds

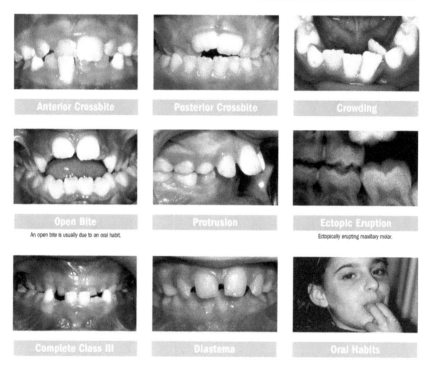

Malocclusions, like those illustrated above, may benefit from early
diagnosis and referral to an orthodontic specialist for a full evaluation.

Figure 2.1

DON'T WAIT FOR A REFERRAL

Many parents rely on their family dentist to tell them when it is time to bring their children in for an orthodontic evaluation. This isn't always a wise strategy, however, because most dentists receive little if any training to identify orthodontic and orthopedic problems in growing children. Most dental offices don't even have the panoramic and cephalometric x-ray equipment needed to identify the many problems that can be prevented or corrected early on, such as impacted or missing teeth.

Every orthodontist I know has a story like the one above, and this is only one story in the many, many cases of patients who have come to me in adulthood with issues that could have been prevented or treated much earlier. If these patients had been referred earlier by their dentist, these problems may have prevented the impaction of adult teeth, or they would have been able to have space maintainers placed for missing teeth that would have saved them thousands of dollars and reduced their time in braces by up to a year. The good news is that you don't need a referral from your family dentist to see an orthodontist. If your child needs orthodontic treatment at an early age, and you have insurance coverage, in almost all instances insurance will cover a large portion of your child's treatment.

NEED FOR EARLY TREATMENT

Take a look back at Figure 2.1 which shows examples of orthodontic problems that should be evaluated, and possibly corrected, at a younger age. If children have one of these problems, early treatment may be necessary. If the orthodontist identifies that the problem should be corrected as early as possible, they will suggest what orthodontists commonly call a "first phase" of treatment. It is called a first phase of treatment because a "second phase" is always needed to straighten the remaining adult teeth that erupt into the mouth, and to correct how the top and bottom teeth bite together. Yes, it is true that when treatment needs to be broken up into two phases like this, it is often considerably more expensive than when treatment can be completed with just one phase of treatment. However, if the child does not receive treatment for a developing problem in a first phase, the cost of treating all the issues after the adult teeth have come in could be not only more expensive, but also take a much longer time and involve surgery, which adds considerably to the overall cost of treatment. With all the above being said, only about 10 percent of children have the types of orthodontic problems that should be corrected at a younger age before all of the adult teeth have come in.[7]

Parents will sometimes ask why braces can't just be added to the adult teeth that come into the mouth as treatment progresses so only one phase of treatment is needed. This is a bad idea because the braces would then need to remain on the teeth for four to five years while waiting for all of the adult teeth to erupt. Leaving braces on the teeth for this long wouldn't be healthy for the teeth because braces are difficult to brush and floss around. It would also substantially increase the number of visits to the orthodontic office to maintain the braces for this long. And anyone who has ever worn braces can tell you that under no circumstances would they want to wear them for that long. Because they are uncomfortable and a nuisance, our goal as orthodontists is to get the best result for our patients while minimizing how long patients are in braces. To achieve this, it is sometimes necessary to stage treatment in two phases. Orthodontists can complete treatment at one time after all of the adult teeth have

---

7   Anthony A. Gianelly, "One-phase versus two-phase treatment," *American Journal of Orthodontics & Dentofacial Orthopedics* 108, no. 5 (1995): 556–559, https://doi.org/10.1016/S0889-5406(95)70057-9

come in as long as there aren't problems that require a first phase of treatment. The good news—this is possible for 90 percent of children.[8]

UNSCRUPULOUS PRACTITIONERS

A concern many parents might have when an orthodontist suggests phase-one treatment for their child is that two phases of treatment may not really be needed and some orthodontists suggest it to most, if not all, of their young patients just to line their pockets with more money. While it is true there are unscrupulous practitioners out there doing this sort of thing, it is obviously not a sustainable way to run an orthodontic practice. Eventually, word would get out that this is going on, and the orthodontic practice would fail due to a lack of patients. Trust is the most important thing in running any business, whether it be an auto repair shop or an orthodontic practice. Verify that your orthodontic practice is certified and practicing orthodontics using the best practice measures by making sure the orthodontist is a member of the American Association of Orthodontists (AAO).

Membership in the AAO signifies the orthodontist has completed four years of dental school and at least two years of residency in a verified residency program.[9] Also, social media and word of mouth recommendations are useful. If most patients at an orthodontic practice are happy with their results and feel like they got prime value for money spent, this is a good sign the orthodontic practice is honest and treating each patient individually using best practices.

---

8   Ibid.

9   Ibid.

RECOGNITION OF HOW ORTHODONTIC PROBLEMS CAN NEGATIVELY IMPACT CHILDREN

If you still are not convinced of the importance of taking your child for an orthodontic consult by age seven, think about the impact that orthodontic issues can have on children and why it is much better to intervene and prevent or treat problems early to avoid bigger problems later. There are three major areas where orthodontic problems can really impact children—speech, health of the teeth and jaws, and self-esteem.

SPEECH PROBLEMS

Perhaps you may not automatically link speech problems with orthodontic issues. However, orthodontic issues—in particular, malocclusions (which is a fancy word for saying that the teeth are not positioned well when the mouth is closed)—can have a strong, negative impact on a child's speech. Teeth positioning plays a critical role in a person's ability to produce sounds, in particular the strident sounds like *t, s, z, f, v, sh, ch, j,* and *zh*. Strident sounds are ones produced with a strong noise; air is forced against the teeth and other parts of the mouth and tongue to produce the sounds. When teeth are not correctly positioned, these sounds are much more difficult to produce, leading to speech problems. In fact, various studies have shown that up to 60 percent of all speech disorders may be caused by malocclusion—and the more severe the malocclusion, the more severe the speech disorder.[10]

---

10 K. M. Leavy, G. J. Cisneros, and E. M. LeBlanc, "Malocclusion and Its Relationship to Speech, Sound Production: Redefining the Effect of Malocclusal Traits on Sounds Production," *Am J Orthod Dentofacial Orthop.* 150, no. 1, (2016): 116–23, https://doi.org/10.1016/j.ajodo.2015.12.015

HEALTH OF THE TEETH AND JAWS

When it comes to the health of the teeth and jaws, early intervention is best. At the age of seven, many adult teeth are beginning to come into the mouth. This is the best time to correct any abnormalities that may be preventing the teeth from coming in, such as extra adult teeth, or baby teeth that aren't falling out like they should. Any crossbites that may be occurring between the top and bottom teeth at this age should be identified and corrected as well to prevent gum recession and damage to the teeth themselves. Also, bad oral habits, such as thumb sucking, should be addressed at this age to prevent jaw growth abnormalities and malpositioning of the teeth. And finally, any breathing and airway problems—that can be caused by things like seasonal allergies and enlarged tonsils—adversely affecting how the jaws are growing should be identified and referred to an Ear, Nose, and Throat (ENT) doctor for evaluation and possible correction.

SELF-ESTEEM

As parents, we all want our children to grow up with a healthy self-esteem. It is important for children to feel confident in who they are and to feel confident in who they can become. As young children, they may not notice or care their teeth are crooked, but as they approach the teenage years, physical appearance may become more important and self-esteem issues may arise as teens navigate through the process of becoming adults. Problems with the appearance of the teeth can strongly affect a teenager's self-esteem. In fact, studies have concluded that there is a strong association between a teenager's unhappiness with how their teeth look and the development of low self-esteem, and that this is particularly true for adolescent girls.[11] There are even studies that show a link between malocclusions in children and adolescents and an increased risk of being bullied.[12]

The importance of problems with self-esteem should not be underestimated, especially in children. Many of these issues may escalate if ignored, leading to depression or even suicide. Nowadays, these problems are exacerbated by the presence of social media, because children can't even escape the bullying they are experiencing at school while at home. It follows them through apps like Facebook, Instagram, and Snapchat. Having teeth with many issues can plague a child's life when it comes to social media—it's very hard to escape embarrassment or shame when camera phones can post a picture online in seconds.

The worst part is, sometimes kids don't want to tell their parents about the bullying either. Maybe it's too embarrassing, or they don't actually want their parents to worry about them too much. So, they end up keeping it bottled up inside. When I was young, I had bad acne and didn't want to talk to my parents about how it was affecting me because I was embarrassed. One day, my dad finally took me to the dermatologist, and I'm glad he did as I was able to dramatically improve my skin. I probably would've just continued to suffer with that problem and let it damage me emotionally if he had not intervened.

---

11   M. H. Jung, "Evaluation of the Effects of Malocclusion and Orthodontic Treatment on Self-Esteem in an Adolescent Population," *Am J Orthod Dentofacial Orthop.* 138, no. 2 (2010): 160-166, https://doi.org/10.1016/j.ajodo.2008.08.040; D. Dhanani and Y. Kaul, "Dental Disorders Impact and Influence on Self-Esteem Levels Among Teenagers," *International Journal of Dental Research and Oral Sciences* 2, no. 1 (2017), https://actascientifica.com/IJDROS/pdf/IJDROS-02-0010.pdf

12   J. Seehra, J. T. Newton and A. T. DiBiase, "Bullying in Schoolchildren – Its Relationship to Dental Appearance and Psychosocial Implications: An Update for GDPs," *British Dental Journal* 210 (2011): 411–15, https://doi.org/10.1038/sj.bdj.2011.339

As an orthodontist, I am primarily concerned with the physical health of my patient's teeth, jaw, and bite. However, having repeatedly witnessed firsthand the emotional effects associated with having poor looking teeth, I know that treating patients' teeth and creating a beautiful smile is just as important for my patients' emotional health as it is for their physical health.

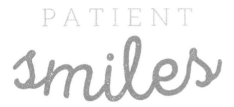

PATIENT *smiles*

What I remember about my childhood is that I was always bullied for my smile; kids called me a horse. I was small with a small face and big teeth; too many teeth for my mouth. I was always ashamed to smile and had no confidence. I wasn't a good student. I couldn't or didn't want to answer questions and was ashamed to talk. So, I didn't do well in school at all.

As I grew older and into my teen years, I knew I really wanted braces to fix my teeth; it was a dream. But, I had to pay for everything out of pocket myself. Neither I, nor my family, had dental insurance. So, I worked hard and saved money and when I turned nineteen, I finally decided to go for it. I found a dental clinic with an orthodontist I could walk to from my parents' home; it just happened to be Dr. Verbic's office. The moment I sat down in the chair, I knew I was in the right place.

Dr. Verbic told me he could definitely give me the smile I wanted, but he strongly suggested that I have four teeth removed . . . four premolars. I trusted him and his knowledge and expertise. But the added cost of removing teeth meant I had to work even harder in order to pay for treatment. I had to trust him that it would be worth it. Dr. Verbic referred me to an oral surgeon and I went for a consultation.

The oral surgeon asked, "Are you sure you want to remove these teeth? You can't get them back."

I told him I was extremely confident in Dr. Verbic's recommendation. The four teeth were removed and the recovery was very simple. In fact, only about a week later, I was in Dr. Verbic's office getting my braces on. I wore these braces for two years and I was a model patient. I was not messing around. I wore my rubber bands as instructed and finished treatment earlier than expected.

From the very moment my treatment started, there were big changes in me and in my life. The fact that I was finally fixing my smile gave me confidence; it propelled me as a student. I started communicating and participating in class. In fact, throughout the rest of my time in treatment I got straight A's in school, and I am about to graduate from college this year. Getting treatment made a huge difference in my life—there are so many things I can accomplish now. I've never felt so confident. Because of my experience and the difference orthodontic treatment made in my life, I decided to major in a predental program in college. When I graduate, I really hope to go on to dental school. I want to be an orthodontist and make a difference in other peoples' lives.

Here is something funny: A few years after my treatment, my predental program required me to shadow a local orthodontist. Guess who I chose? That's right: Dr. Verbic. Now, I get the chance to watch as he treats and interacts with patients. My dream is to help people in the same way Dr. Verbic helped not only me, but so many other people. Orthodontic treatment has really changed the trajectory of my life and, for that, I am so grateful. It was worth every hard-earned penny. **—WANDA N.**

As you can see, there are many good reasons to seek an orthodontic evaluation for your child around the age of seven. These reasons range from evaluating orthodontic concerns to intervene early and avoid more invasive treatment later, to addressing self-esteem issues a child may be having due to teasing about the appearance of his or her teeth. Addressing these issues early is best for the child; just ask Mary, the patient I referred to earlier who lost a baby tooth at age thirty.

chapter three

STRAIGHTENING SMILES IN ADULTS

It wasn't too many years ago when the image that popped into your head when you heard the word *braces* was probably of a teenager with a mouth full of metal. Getting braces was often a rite of passage during the teenage years. However, as we discovered in the last chapter, treatment often begins in children before they are even teenagers. At the other end of the spectrum, there are also more and more adults seeking orthodontic treatment today.

One question I'm asked all the time is, "Am I too old to get braces?" And the short answer is no. No one is ever too old to get braces. In fact, one of my oldest patients was ninety-three years old when she started orthodontic treatment—I am not joking. As techniques and technology for treatment continues to develop, costs come down, and orthodontic treatment becomes available to more people, the door has opened for many adults who, for one reason or another, did not or could not get orthodontic treatment when they were younger.

In fact, the number of adult patients has increased so much that 25 percent of orthodontic patients today are adults. According to the AAO, the number of adult patients increased 14 percent between 2010 and 2012, resulting in the treatment of more than 1.2 million adults over age eighteen.[13] Another huge jump in orthodontic treatment is in adult male patients. In 2012, the number of adult male patients was 44 percent of all adult patients, which was a 29 percent increase from 2010. There has been such a huge increase in the number of adults seeking orthodontic treatment the AAO created an Adult Hall of Fame page on their website that highlights the stories of adult patients seeking orthodontic treatment.

The number of adult patients keeps growing. There are several reasons for this, including the "my teeth weren't that bad as a child, but I really want to fix them now" reason; the "my family couldn't afford braces for me when I was a child" reason; and the "there are so many better treatment options available today" reason. Oh, and there is a fourth reason: "I had braces when I was a teenager, but didn't wear my retainer as instructed and my teeth shifted."

REASONS FOR GROWTH IN ADULT ORTHODONTIC TREATMENT

Orthodontic treatment was once reserved for children whose teeth were in the worst condition, those who had the most crowding or largest overbites. When I was in grade school and junior high back in the 1980s, the children with the most-obvious orthodontic problems had braces. But over the last three decades, more and more parents saw how braces could benefit their children for the rest of their lives.

---

13 "Adult Hall of Fame Celebrates Professionals Getting Orthodontic Treatment," American Association of Orthodontists, www.aaoinfo.org/news/2014/04/adult-hall-fame-celebrates-professionals-getting-orthodontic-treatment

They also began seeking treatment for their children with less-obvious problems and for themselves.

ESTABLISHED BENEFIT OF TREATING MILD-TO-MODERATE ORTHODONTIC PROBLEMS

Today, parents understand the benefits of treating even mild-to-moderate malocclusions in their children's teeth. As adults, people are choosing treatment for themselves for lots of different reasons. They may work in a high-profile profession or one in which they interact daily with hundreds or people and their smile is the first thing people see. Some may feel that having crooked teeth is holding them back professionally or personally. Some may have an important life event coming up and want to look their absolute best for it. Some may feel self-conscious about their smile, rarely show their teeth, and want to feel more confident; or they are starting out on their own in a new stage of life and want to improve their smile and self-confidence. Other reasons may be that they have difficulty keeping their crooked teeth clean, have been fighting cavities their whole life, and know having straight teeth will lead to overall better dental and gum health. Some people have spent a good portion of their lives hiding their teeth and finally have decided to stop hiding. Or, in some cases, some people had teeth that were straight throughout childhood and adolescence, but, in adulthood, their teeth have shifted due to injury or tooth loss.

REDUCED COST

Many families couldn't afford braces for their children when they were growing up, especially if their children's teeth weren't that bad. As these children have grown up, costs have decreased and insurance options, health savings accounts (HSAs), and financing have increased payment options for treatment. This has made treatment more affordable for these adults now paying for themselves (in addition to parents paying for their children today). Adults who can now afford to pay for their own treatment are often choosing to fix issues they have put up with for years. For adults, seeking and purchasing orthodontic treatment is often a much more emotional experience, compared to parents paying for their child's treatment on a need basis. Adult patients know what it feels like to grow up with crooked teeth. They have strong feelings about how having orthodontic problems affected their life and will often talk about what they went through before seeking treatment. The decision to pay for orthodontic treatment is often very personal and emotional.

NEW TECHNOLOGY

A third reason for the increase in adult patients undergoing orthodontic treatment is the advent of and continued improvement in aligner technology, such as Invisalign, and the development of ceramic braces. Adults can sometimes be opposed to wearing braces because they are afraid of what others will think about an adult having a mouth full of metal. Invisalign has effectively resolved this worry by eliminating the need for traditional braces in a growing number of adult patients. We will spend a whole chapter on Invisalign later in the book, but this technology has truly revolutionized orthodontic treatment and has encouraged thousands of new patients to seek treatment. This treatment option is far less invasive, much easier to use, and results in great patient outcomes.

However, there are still patients who are not good candidates for Invisalign, contrary to Invisalign's online self-assessment tool. The number of patients who are not good candidates is shrinking every year due to advances in the understanding of how teeth move with clear aligners, and engineering improvements to the aligner systems themselves. Still, if you are an adult who has gone to several orthodontists for an opinion and the consensus is that you should have treatment with braces, keep in mind what matters most is the result, not how you get there. If you would rather have Invisalign but have been told you would get a better result with braces, consider that the time you spend in treatment will be insignificant compared to the time you will have to live with a result you are not happy with. Also, ask yourself how you feel about other adults around your age who are wearing braces. Do they look silly to you? Or do you feel happy for them that they are undergoing treatment to feel better about themselves and to improve their lives? If braces are recommended for you or your child and you really hate the idea of the traditional metal mouth, ceramic braces are a good option. Some orthodontic offices charge a bit more for them, but they are clear and not as noticeable as traditional braces.

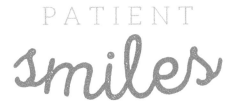

PATIENT *smiles*

Back in the 1960s, I wore braces and it seemed like no other teenagers had them. I hated them! People made fun of me and I felt like having braces was ruining my social life. I told my parents I wanted them off and, surprisingly, they said okay (I am still shocked they agreed!). So, the orthodontist took them off and gave me a retainer, which, of course, I didn't wear. Well, as I got older, there was one tooth that was very crooked and it really, really bothered me. I complained and talked about fixing it for years, but there was no way I was going to wear braces again. Then, around 1999, I heard about Invisalign and thought, this is perfect for me! But I still didn't go for a consultation. Something was always getting in the way ... moving, my own teenagers in braces, and on and on. After years of complaining and talking about my annoying crooked tooth, my husband turned to me one day last year and said, "Just go get it fixed!" So, I did! I went for an orthodontic consultation, was told I was a good candidate for Invisalign and started treatment last September. No one even knew I was wearing Invisalign. I wore the trays exactly as instructed … twenty-two hours a day. Yes, it was somewhat inconvenient (because I couldn't eat or drink certain things with them on), but it was so easy and I only had to go to the orthodontist every six to eight weeks after the first couple of months. I finished treatment just a few weeks ago in the middle of July—just in time for my daughter's wedding! Fixing my teeth took less than one year! It's great! It is hard to believe I waited so long, but, finally, at sixty-six years old, my crooked, annoying tooth is perfectly straight and I am so happy. —SUSAN L.

If you are an adult who wore braces as a teenager, but you have experienced relapse or unwanted movement of teeth (i.e., didn't follow instructions on wearing your retainer), then orthodontic re-treatment generally takes a relatively short amount of time. This is because teeth almost never relapse fully back to the positions they were in prior to orthodontic treatment. In most cases, simple realignment with aligners such as Invisalign can re-create a perfectly straight smile. Most adults will experience relapse with crowding on the lower front teeth. Orthodontists have identified this as the most unstable area in patients and many have gone to using fixed retainers to prevent this most common form of relapse.

SPECIAL CONSIDERATIONS FOR ADULT PATIENTS

So, yes, there is a large influx in the treatment of adult patients, but there *are* some special considerations for adults seeking orthodontic treatment. One of these considerations is the health of the teeth and supporting structures, such as the gums and the bone that holds the teeth in the jaws. The teeth and supporting structures must be in good health before orthodontic treatment can begin. This is because orthodontic treatment involves the manipulation of the teeth within the gum tissue and jaw bone. Light stress is placed on these structures to move the teeth into the correct position. Adding stress to unhealthy tissue and bone will lead to pain, worsening of any disease, and, of course, the orthodontic treatment would be ineffective. Therefore, the patient must be cavity-free, and any periodontal disease must be under control before the braces are placed or treatment with Invisalign can begin.

Another consideration for adult treatment is that if there are missing teeth, treatment can generally take a little longer. When teeth are missing, the remaining teeth surrounding the tooth that was removed can drift into the space of the missing tooth. This "drifting" of teeth takes weeks to months to occur, so if you plan on replacing missing teeth with bridges or implants you are better off doing so sooner than later. If accomplished within a few weeks of a tooth being removed, orthodontic treatment can often be avoided altogether. The longer you wait, the more the surrounding teeth can drift into the space of the missing tooth. And the more drifting that occurs, the longer orthodontic treatment can take. In cases of severe drifting, when patients want to replace missing teeth, treatment can sometimes take up to three years to finish.

There really are only a few considerations that make getting orthodontic treatment different for an adult compared to a child or adolescent. If your teeth and gums are healthy, then you can start treatment whether you are thirty-four years old, sixty-two years old, or even ninety-three years old. We are living longer and, thanks to great general dental care and improved oral hygiene, we are keeping our teeth as we age. Why not have a great smile when you are a hundred years old?

chapter four

PATIENCE LEADS TO A BEAUTIFUL SMILE: TYPICAL LENGTH OF TIME FOR ORTHODONTIC TREATMENT

In an era of instant gratification, the length of time it can take to complete orthodontic treatment is a major concern and sometimes even a deterrent to getting the smile you've always dreamed of.

But it shouldn't be.

Out of the thousands of patients I have treated, not a single one has told me they regretted their decision. Quite the contrary. I have patients return to me years later and say that getting braces was the best thing they ever did for themselves or, in the case of children, they say it was the best thing their parents did for them.

Really, a more accurate way to think about straightening your teeth is to ask yourself the question, "How much longer am I going to allow my crooked teeth to hold me back in life ... to prevent me from living to my full potential?" But you shouldn't take my word for it. After all, I'm an orthodontist and I have a financial incentive to convince you that braces or Invisalign are the best thing since sliced bread, right? Instead, you should probably ask someone you know who has had orthodontic treatment. I'd be very surprised, however, if they told you anything different.

For your reference, the average amount of time it takes to finish orthodontic treatment these days is twenty months. This is based on data from thousands of orthodontic patients across the United States.[14] I always use this data as a starting point with every new patient. But, this number is just a data point. There are lots of factors that influence the actual length of treatment time in braces or Invisalign for each individual patient.

FACTORS THAT INFLUENCE TREATMENT TIME

The first factor is one that will lead to increased time in braces or Invisalign. This is how severe the malocclusion and misalignment of the teeth are to begin with. Unfortunately, this factor is one that neither you nor I as an orthodontist can control. Patients with severe orthodontic problems will usually take longer to complete treatment than patients with mild problems. Some conditions that can lengthen treatment are impacted teeth, severely rotated teeth, severe spacing, severe crowding, a large overbite or underbite, and extra or missing teeth.

But there is good news. Even if you have one of the more severe orthodontic problems, there are many additional factors that lead to reduced treatment time and these factors are ones a qualified orthodontist can control.

---

14   Aliki Tsichlaki et al., "How long does treatment with fixed orthodontic appliances last? A systematic review," *American Journal of Orthodontics & Dentofacial Orthopedics* 149, no. 3 (2016): 308–318, https://doi.org/10.1016/j.ajodo.2015.09.020

A well-designed treatment plan that incorporates efficient treatment methodology, a highly-trained staff, and an efficient system in place in the orthodontic office are essential factors that influence treatment time and patient compliance.

In addition, there are newer technological advances in orthodontics that can decrease treatment time. For example, there are effective surgical techniques available that, when used in conjunction with braces or Invisalign, can cut treatment time by 20–40 percent. However, these techniques also drive up the overall cost significantly. These techniques include corticotomy (more invasive) and piezocision (less invasive).[15] The description for how these techniques work is very technical, but basically, an oral surgeon makes small cuts into the gum line and into the underlying bone to stimulate the bone. This bone stimulation allows for pronounced and faster tooth movement within the bone within a window of time (up to six months) post-surgery. Also on the market are intraoral vibration devices, which are FDA approved, but their effectiveness is not as proven scientifically (i.e., few clinical studies). The vibration techniques are not invasive and work by applying vibration to the teeth (after the braces or Invisalign are on the teeth) for about twenty minutes per day; this vibration is thought to stimulate the bone and promote faster movement of the teeth.

---

15   Jorge Cano et al., "Corticotomy-Assisted Orthodontics," *J Clin Exp Dent.* 4, no. 1 (2012): e54–e59, https://doi.org/10.4317/jced.50642; Jean David M. Sebaoun, Jérôme Surmenian, and Serge Dibart, "Accelerated Orthodontic Treatments with Piezocision: A Mini-Invasive Alternative to Alveolar Corticotomies," *Orthod. Fr* 82 (2011): 311-19, https://doi.org/10.1051/orthodfr/2011142; Flavio Uribe et al., "Patients', Parents', and Orthodontists' Perceptions of the Need for and Costs of Additional Procedures to Reduce Treatment Time," *Am J Orthod Dentofacial Orthop* 145, no. 4 (2014): S65–73, https://doi.org/10.1016/j.ajodo.2013.12.015; Abdullah M. Aldrees, "Do Customized Orthodontic Appliances and Vibration Devices Provide More Efficient Treatment Than Conventional Methods?" *Korean J Orthodon.* 46, no. 3 (2016): 180–85, https://doi.org/10.4041/kjod.2016.46.3.180

However, when I explain what is involved with the surgical techniques and the added cost of using them, most of my patients say, "No thanks, we're ok with treatment lasting a bit longer." I also tell interested patients about the adjunct vibration technique, but because this adds significantly to the cost of treatment and it is still a new treatment with not a lot of data to back up its effectiveness, again, most of my patients opt to go the more-traditional route.

FOUR PILLARS OF ORTHODONTIC TREATMENT

In addition to all the factors a qualified orthodontist and staff can control, the most important ones known to reduce treatment time are *all* ones you as a patient can control. They are all free and easy to implement and can more than make up for the added treatment time of the things you cannot control. I call these factors "the four pillars of orthodontic treatment." And I call them pillars because they are that important. Not only do they lead to much shorter treatment times, but they also lead to much better results. The opposite is also true. Failure to follow the four pillars of orthodontic treatment results in increased treatment time. There was a study published based on a review of 140 comprehensive orthodontic patient records from five different orthodontic practices in the United States. The data revealed that treatment time was significantly increased due to the following patient controlled factors in missed appointments, broken/loose brackets and bands, and poor oral hygiene.[16]

As an orthodontist, I create a customized plan for each of my patients. I know exactly what to do to fix his or her teeth and will follow my plan down to each tiny wire, bracket, and rubber band

---

16   F. R. Beckwith, et al., "An Evaluation of Factors Affecting Duration of Orthodontic Treatment," *Am J Orthod Dentofacial Orthop* 115, no. 4 (1999): 439–47, accessed at www.ncbi.nlm.nih.gov/pubmed/10194290

and its role in moving the teeth to create that perfect smile. But, I can do everything right and treatment could still take half the time or even double the time of the twenty-two-month average treatment time. Why? Because the length of treatment is very, very dependent on whether or not my patient follows the directions I give (the four pillars). It really is up to the patient. Those who follow the four pillars may finish their treatment in twelve to fourteen months; those who don't may be looking at up to four years in braces!

—DR. VERBIC

FIRST PILLAR – KEEP YOUR APPOINTMENTS

The first pillar is to always keep your appointments. Researchers found that for each missed appointment, an extra month of treatment time was required.[17] So, you can see why it is so important to keep your appointments.

The number of times you must visit your orthodontist for adjustments can vary, but the average patient will need fifteen appointments to complete treatment with braces. This can be a real challenge with how busy our lives have become in this day and age. A good strategy is to find a day and time of the week that consistently works for you. For instance, if you are usually free on Mondays afternoons at three o'clock, then you should try to always schedule your appointments on this day and time. It will help you remember your appointments if they are always on the same day and time. If you have multiple children in treatment, or if you are in treatment at the same time as your children, you should try to schedule all your appointments at the same time. This will reduce the number of trips you make back and forth to the office. If possible, you should try to make your appointments between 9 a.m. and 3 p.m. This can be challenging as

---

17   Ibid.

most people are at work or school during these hours, but because most people have school and work obligations during these hours, it is not a coincidence that orthodontic practices are not as busy during these hours. Because most orthodontists and their staff are less busy during these hours, they can usually get more done on patients that come in during these times, and this may lead to fewer visits for adjustments. Some practices even offer discounts for patients that can come in during these slower-than-normal hours of the day.

If you must miss an appointment, try to reschedule it as soon as possible. Most practices have software that can automatically send appointment reminders via text, email, or voicemail. If you miss your appointment, they will usually call you back to try to reschedule to keep your overall treatment time on track. Despite our best efforts though, all orthodontists have their stories about patients who come in once every six months for their adjustment appointments. Nothing good usually happens when patients wait this long between appointments ... so don't be *that* patient.

SECOND PILLAR – MAINTAIN YOUR ORAL HYGIENE

Maintaining good oral hygiene means brushing and flossing throughout treatment and after. Poor oral hygiene leads to cavities, and if a cavity requires treatment while braces are on the teeth, it will often require the temporary removal of some of the braces so a dentist can do a filling. It can take one to three months to realign a tooth that has had its brace removed. In rare cases, when cavities become severe, they can require more-extensive treatment, such as root canals and/or crowns. This can delay orthodontic treatment even longer. Under the worst circumstances, a tooth may require extraction, which can delay treatment many months. Poor oral hygiene may also lead to swelling of the gums (gingivitis), which can make it difficult to position braces properly on teeth and can make it difficult if not impossible to close gaps or spaces between teeth. Hardened plaque (tartar) can also prevent gaps and spaces from fully closing. When poor oral hygiene habits are prolonged, they can lead to periodontitis, which may make it necessary to suspend orthodontic treatment until a deep cleaning is performed and a patient can demonstrate the ability to consistently keep the teeth clean.

THIRD PILLAR – WATCH WHAT YOU EAT

It goes without saying that braces and Invisalign aligners must stay on the teeth for the teeth to move, which brings us to the third pillar of treatment. When patients first get their braces, especially children, it can be difficult adjusting to foods that will not break off the braces. Orthodontists typically advise patients to avoid eating hard foods, such as Italian bread, apples, and nuts. But, in reality, patients may continue eating all the foods they enjoy; they just have to eat them differently. The golden rule is to eat foods in smaller bites. For example, cut apples up into smaller pieces instead of biting into a whole apple. Don't eat corn on the cob—remove the corn from the cob first and then eat it. Cut carrots into smaller pieces instead of biting off a chunk of a whole carrot. Braces are put onto the teeth with an intermediate strength adhesive, so they won't come off with careful eating. They can also be removed easily without damaging enamel when the treatment is finished. A stronger adhesive would allow patients to eat hard foods however they wanted, but this would risk damage to enamel upon removal of the braces. The only person who would be happy with this scenario would be the dentist who places veneers. With orthodontic adhesives that are currently used, damage to healthy enamel never occurs. Another common way braces are broken off teeth is when children bite on pencils or pens at school. No matter how the braces are broken off the teeth, it can add one to two months to the overall treatment time each and every time it happens. In much the same way that broken braces can extend treatment time, when patients do not wear their Invisalign aligners for the recommended twenty-two to twenty-four hours per day, treatment time is extended. When the aligners are worn fewer than twenty-two hours per day, the teeth will not move where they are supposed to. If this happens, then the orthodontist will have to order more aligners to achieve the desired outcome, and the result is a longer treatment time.

FOURTH PILLAR – WEAR YOUR ELASTICS

The fourth and final pillar of orthodontic treatment is one that usually causes treatment to extend much longer than it needs to and causes the most headache with orthodontists and parents alike. In the later stages of orthodontic treatment, patients are instructed to wear elastics (dreaded rubber bands) to correct how the top teeth bite with the bottom teeth. But some patients, especially teenagers, do not always follow instructions. If you are a parent with a teen in braces, I assume you are already aware of this phenomenon.

Each top tooth has a certain shape to it that fits with each bottom tooth in the same way jigsaw puzzle pieces fit together. This is often referred to as the "occlusion" by dentists and orthodontists. In the past, it was thought that if teeth did not fit together properly it would cause pain and degeneration in the jaw points or the teeth themselves. Through decades of research, however, this was shown not to be the case for most people.[18] Today, orthodontists strive to achieve a correct bite to improve the appearance of the smile in severe cases such as a large overbite or underbite, and to prevent unwanted movement or relapse of the teeth after treatment is completed. Empirical evidence shows substantially less unwanted tooth movement with a corrected bite than with a bite that has not been corrected.

That being said, adequate use of retainers after orthodontic treatment will prevent unwanted movement of teeth anyway. So why do orthodontists strive to correct bites with elastics for patients with mild overbites or underbites that do *not* adversely affect the appearance of the smile? As orthodontists, we know patients are not always good about wearing retainers. We want our patients to have the best possible chance of keeping their smiles beautiful for the rest of their lives and to avoid having to go through orthodontic treatment again in the future. So, we strive to achieve a correct bite even when it adds to the overall treatment time when patients do not adhere to wearing the elastics as prescribed. Keep in mind that orthodontic elastics are powerful. Most patients' bites can be corrected within three months by wearing the elastics twenty-four hours a day, seven days a week. But if you get tired of battling your child to wear the elastics and the smile is straight and beautiful, just let your orthodontist know. Braces are not a prison for the teeth and there are no adverse health

---

18   Cyril Sadowsky and Alan M. Polson, "Temporomanidublar Disorders and Functional Occlusion after Orthodontic Treatment: Results of Two Long-Term Studies," *Am J Orthod* 86, no. 5 (1984): 386–90, https://doi.org/10.1016/S0002-9416(84)90030-7; D. Manfredini et al., "Dental Occlusion, Body Posture, and Temporomandibular Disorders: Where We Are Now and Where We Are Heading For," *J Oral Rehabilitation* 39, no. 6 (2012): 463–71, https://doi.org/10.1111/j.1365-2842.2012.02291.x ; D. Gesch, O. Bernhardt and A. Kirbschus, "Association of Malocclusion and Functional Occlusion with Temporomandibular Disorders (TMD) in Adults: A Systematic Review of Population-Based Studies," *Quintessence International* 35, no. 3 (2004): 211–21, https://www.ncbi.nlm.nih.gov/pubmed/15119680

consequences to having an imperfect bite. However, if you or your child want a perfect bite, elastics would be the route to get there. We want our patients and their parents to be happy, and if it means removing the braces even though the bite is not absolutely correct, it is certainly not the end of the world. Just make sure you (or your child) are faithful about wearing your retainers and your smile will stay beautiful forever. The only people that will know your bite is not ideal are your dentist and your orthodontist. We'll keep it our little secret.

The end result: if you are being seen by a qualified orthodontist who has a well-trained staff and they are using a well-developed, efficient treatment plan designed specifically for you, *and* you do your part and follow the guidelines outlined in the four pillars, you could finish treatment in twelve to eighteen months or less.

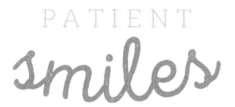
PATIENT *smiles*

It all started when I noticed in pictures how much my teeth had moved since I had braces at fourteen years old. I had stopped wearing a retainer in my twenties and my teeth had moved so much. I didn't like how my teeth looked at all, so I made a decision to do something about it. After talking with Dr. Verbic, who presented me with the option of braces or Invisalign, I chose braces because I felt that it would be the fastest route for me—I wouldn't have the option to take them out, forget to wear them, etc. I was very comfortable with the look of clear brackets because they allowed me to feel comfortable and still look professional at work.

I committed to the treatment plan given to me, which I think is very important. You have to be diligent and committed to the treatment and care plan provided by the office. They are the experts and they know what is going to get you to your end goal. I knew if I followed their guidelines, I would meet or beat the timeline to de-band. Dr. Verbic felt it would take twelve months if I kept timely appointments and was committed to wearing and changing the prescribed rubber bands. I did exactly what he said and he was right. However, I was always prepared to wear them longer, if it meant getting the result we wanted. I am truly happy with the experience and my results. —BRYNNEN.C.

PITFALLS OF INSTANT GRATIFICATION

This is where we need to talk again about our culture of instant gratification. Often people fall into the trap of wanting something right away. They have a wedding or a big beach vacation coming up soon and want perfect teeth for all the photos. Or, they have finally decided to fix their teeth and just want it done as quickly and as cheaply as possible. Well, unfortunately, there are a lot of businesses out there that prey on peoples' quest for instant gratification.

Currently, there are true internet scams with the aim of convincing people they can use DIY (Do It Yourself) braces. There are videos or tutorials that provide instruction on how to use elastic bands to close gaps in their teeth. This is a terrible idea and can lead to serious damage and even loss of teeth.[19] There is also a new trend involving mail-order orthodontics. This is a type of online "orthodontic service" in which the service decides if you are a good candidate by evaluating a selfie of your teeth that you send to them. Then, the service sends you a kit for you to make an impression mold of your teeth. You mail this mold back and they determine your treatment based on it. You then pay (up to about $2,000) and they send you the orthodontic appliance (clear aligners like Invisalign) to use on your teeth. Yikes. Mail-order orthodontics is not a good idea. It could lead to loss of

---

19   "Consumers Cautioned about 'DIY' Orthodontic Treatment," Consumer Alert, American Association of Orthodontists, https://www.aaoinfo.org/

money with no good result at best, and harm to your teeth and gums at worst. It's important to be seen in person by a licensed orthodontist who can truly evaluate your jaw, gums, and teeth and determine the best treatment for your unique, individual orthodontic situation.

Beware of scams and unscrupulous companies like these. There is a reason orthodontists spend many years—first in dental school and then in orthodontic residency school—learning all about teeth and how to evaluate and treat dental disorders and how to use orthodontic appliances to move teeth safely and correctly. There are lots of things you can DIY; moving your teeth is *not* one of them.

In addition, there are general dentists out there who are looking to make a lot of money and get in on the orthodontic action by offering people a perfect smile in seven months or less. I get the attraction. Six months versus a potential twenty-two months is a big difference. But here's the thing (time for some clichés): some things are too good to be true. You get what you pay for, so don't believe everything you hear. While this may be safer than the DIY and mail-order braces discussed above, here are the facts. These types of treatments are mass produced in an orthodontic lab, which then sends the braces already "set-up" to dentists to use on their patients. The dentist then just bonds the braces to the teeth in preprogrammed positions and using only one wire. These types of treatments, which often cost almost as much money as traditional braces or Invisalign, don't address any underlying bite problems, which leads to much less stability of the teeth in the jaw and a much-increased chance for teeth to shift once the braces come off. This means the probability of needing future treatment is much higher. Dentists who are selling these types of systems won't explain this to their patients because it is obviously counterproductive to their financial bottom lines. So, do your research, get a second opinion and think carefully about the importance of quality in treating something as important as your teeth.

> *Sometimes, patients come to me and say, "I have heard about these really quick treatment times for braces. Can you do this?" I always tell them that, sure, I can straighten their teeth in six months, but there are big drawbacks to this type of treatment. Without a doubt, 100 percent of the patients I talk to tell me they want their treatment done correctly after I explain the process to them.*
>
> **—DR. VERBIC**

chapter five

FROM CROSSBITES TO CROWDING: COMMON ORTHODONTIC PROBLEMS

We have arrived at the chapter where I will explain in detail some of the orthodontic problems I see in my office. All of the problems included in this chapter are common. This means a lot of children and adults have these problems; therefore, if you or your child has one of these problems ... welcome to the club.

> *I want to state right up front before getting into the details that I've never had a patient with an orthodontic problem I couldn't treat. It's true; I'm not trying to brag. It's simple, really. If a patient is open to both orthodontics and surgery, then I can always come up with a treatment plan and, working together with my team and the patient, we can always arrive at a good result. It's only when patients put restrictions on treatment that results are not optimal.*

> *So, the problems discussed below might look difficult to treat but,*
> *rest assured, all of them can be treated and fixed.*
>
> ### —DR. VERBIC

CROSSBITES

In a healthy bite, all of the upper teeth should overlap the lower teeth in the front and in the back. A crossbite results when this does not happen. There are two types of crossbites: anterior and posterior.

ANTERIOR CROSSBITES

When the lower teeth overlap the upper teeth in the front, they are considered to be an "anterior crossbite." Crossbites on the front teeth can be caused by genetically crowed teeth or by trauma to baby teeth, prior to the adult teeth coming into the mouth. Crossbites on the front teeth should be corrected as early as possible because of the possibility of gum recession that can result. In Figure 5.1a, you can see gum recession on the lower front tooth. The lower tooth looks longer than the others because this is the tooth experiencing gum recession due to the crossbite. The lower tooth is being forced forward by the upper tooth, and the gum and bone underneath the gum that holds the lower tooth in the jaw cannot withstand this force. If left untreated, the health of this tooth will deteriorate. It will likely be lost early in adulthood due to a lack of its supporting structures of bone and gums. However, if corrected early in childhood, the recession is unlikely to get worse and may even regenerate after the tooth is properly positioned out of crossbite as shown below in a before and after treatment photo (see Figures 5.1a, 5.1b).

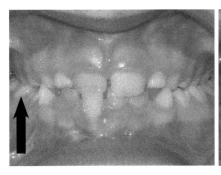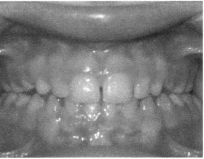

Figures 5.1a, 5.1b

Even when recession is not seen with crossbites on the front teeth, they should be corrected early due to the high probability that recession will occur. Anterior crossbites are typically corrected with braces placed on both the upper and lower teeth.

POSTERIOR CROSSBITES

When the lower teeth overlap the upper teeth in the back, this is termed: "posterior crossbite." Posterior crossbites can have both genetic and environmental causes. Environmental causes include a constricted airway either caused by seasonal allergies or enlarged tonsils, or a thumb-sucking habit. The bone and gums on the back teeth are typically stronger than that on the front teeth, so recession is not typically seen on the back teeth like it is when there is a crossbite on the front teeth. Nevertheless, posterior crossbites should be corrected as early as possible, typically with upper and lower braces or with expanders. If left untreated, posterior crossbites can lead to asymmetrical facial growth. The later in life posterior crossbites are corrected, the less predictable and less stable the correction is, and correction in adulthood can sometimes require upper jaw surgery.

An example of a posterior crossbite correction from my practice is shown below (see Figure 5.2a, and 5.2b).

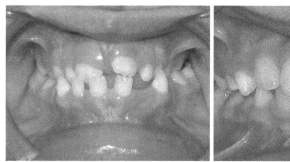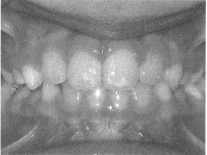

Figure 5.2a and 5.2b

OPEN BITES

Open bites are characterized by front teeth that do not touch. Open bites are caused either by oral habits, such as thumb sucking, or by genetics. If they are caused by oral habits, it is important to work hard to help your child break the habit as soon as possible (see below for a discussion about this). When stopped early enough, the bite will usually close some of the way back together on its own. If needed, braces can be used to close the bite fully after the remaining adult teeth have come into the mouth.

When open bites are caused by genetics, it is much more difficult to correct, and the problem should be addressed as early as possible for the best chance at orthopedic correction. Options to close the bite at an early age, or at least control it from getting worse, include head gear or intra-oral appliances, such as a bionator. It should be noted that some open bites with a genetic cause cannot be adequately controlled or corrected with orthodontic or orthopedic treatment alone. Some severe cases do indeed require surgical correction. An example of a child who was developing an open bite and was treated successfully in my practice is shown below (see Figure 5.3a and 5.3b).

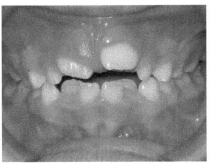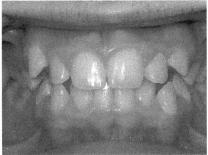

Figures 5.3a and 5.3b

THE THUMB-SUCKING HABIT

We talked about bad habits earlier in chapter one. Now you can see the orthodontic issues, such as crossbites and open bites, that can result if these habits aren't stopped early enough. Ideally, oral habits such as thumb or finger sucking should be stopped by no later than age five to avoid adverse changes to the position of the jaws and teeth. If stopped by the age of five or so, orthodontic treatment can usually be avoided.

Sometimes, getting children to stop sucking their thumb can be very difficult; most parents with children who have a thumb-sucking habit know this all too well. For it to stop, the child really has to want to stop. If the child doesn't want to stop, then most efforts to get him or her to do so will fail. For the most part, social pressures in preschool, kindergarten, and grade school usually contribute to the child stopping on his or her own. If your son or daughter is around friends who aren't sucking their thumbs and your son or daughter still is, they'll feel an immense social pressure to stop the habit. When these habits persist past the age of five or so, it is usually just happening at night while sleeping because social pressure prevents the child from thumb sucking during the day. Thumb or finger sucking sometimes persists at night before bed because it is comforting and helps the child fall asleep.

However, there are some things parents can do to encourage their children to stop sucking their thumbs at night. One idea is to put Band-Aids over the thumbs to help remind children not to suck their thumbs. Positive reinforcement, such as extra bedtime stories or extra time to play video or board games in exchange for not sucking their thumb, can also help. Fun sticker charts to mark the days of no thumb sucking, combined with special rewards, such as a trip to the park or a favorite restaurant for several days in a row of no thumb sucking, are also good ideas. I would advise against putting hot pepper on their thumbs or placing socks over their hands, as this can appear to children to be a punishment. When children feel like they are being punished for sucking their thumbs, they won't stop the behavior, parents will get stressed out and the cycle will continue.

SEVERE CROWDING

Severe crowding of the teeth is exactly what it sounds like. There are too many teeth in too small a space (Figure 5.4). Crowding usually has a genetic origin, but may also be caused by the early loss of baby teeth that act as space maintainers for the adult teeth that replace them. When severe crowding of teeth in either the upper or lower jaw is identified and treated early enough, then the need for the removal of adult teeth can be minimized. In these cases, severely crowed teeth are treated with braces or expanders or a combination of the two. Some orthodontists will recommend against treating crowed teeth early and will instead recommend extractions of select adult teeth after all the adult teeth have come into the mouth. This is a decision parents should make in consultation with their orthodontist. Please see chapter nine for a more-detailed discussion about the removal of adult teeth.

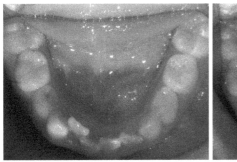
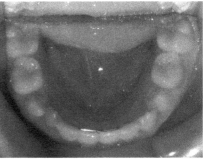

Figures 5.4a and 5.4b

PROTRUSION OF UPPER TEETH

Protrusion of upper teeth, or what is commonly called a large overbite, is genetic and is usually due to a small lower jaw. Research indicates that correction of the protrusion at an early age can reduce the risk of injury to the upper front teeth. Therefore, some parents in consultation with their orthodontist will choose to correct this condition at an early age, prior to all of the adult teeth coming into the mouth. Braces on the upper teeth are usually used to correct the protrusion. However, it is possible to treat this in one phase after all of the adult teeth are in. The patient shown below (Figure 5.5a and 5.5b) chose to have orthodontic treatment in my practice after all the adult teeth had erupted so treatment could be completed in a single phase.

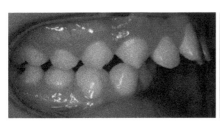
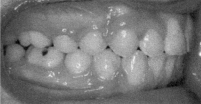

Figures 5.5a and 5.5b

DEEP BITES

Deep bites occur when there is too much overlap of the upper front teeth with the lower front teeth. They usually have a genetic cause. With the teeth biting this way, the upper front teeth can damage the gums of the lower front teeth. The lower front teeth may also damage the gums of the upper front teeth on the palate. If your child has a similar bite, you will want to get an orthodontic exam to find out if phase 1 orthodontic treatment is needed. If it is, your orthodontist will usually move the front teeth out of this poor biting relationship and give your child a special retainer to wear, such as a bionator or Hawley retainer with a bite plate, to prevent the teeth from moving back into a deep bite. As is the case with crossbites on the front teeth, some regeneration of gum tissue can occur if the condition is diagnosed and treated at an early age. Figures 5.6a and 5.6b below show a child with a deep bite in my practice that did not have any damage to his gums. Orthodontic treatment was, therefore, delayed until all of his adult teeth were in his mouth so it could be completed in a single phase.

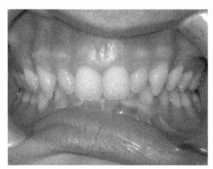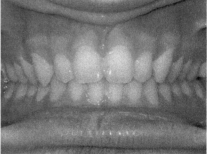

Figures 5.6a and 5.6b

UNDERBITES

Underbites, or class III malocclusions, occur when most or all of the front teeth are in crossbite. They are usually indications that the lower jaw is growing larger and out of proportion to the upper jaw. This condition has a strong genetic component and typically runs in the family. Your orthodontist may ask if you or your spouse had an underbite, or if there is anyone else in the family with an underbite. The condition should be addressed at an early age and prior to all of the adult teeth coming into the mouth. Research has shown that if this condition is not severe, it can be corrected with orthopedic facemask therapy, which involves the child wearing a facemask, as shown below in Figure 5.7, in order to aid the upper jaw to grow further forward so it is proportional to the lower jaw and the teeth are not in crossbite.

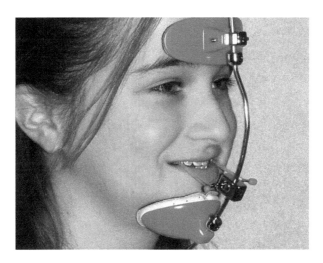

Figure 5.7

It is important to note this condition typically gets more severe as the child grows, but no orthodontist can predict precisely the extent of future growth. In severe cases, jaw surgery in combination with orthodontic treatment may be required after the child is done growing. Females typically stop growing around seventeen years of age, whereas males stop growing around twenty-two years of age. Your orthodontist can use x-rays to check if growth is complete. An example mild class III correction with a facemask in my practice is shown below (see Figure 5.8a and 5.8b).

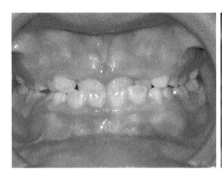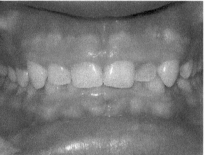

Figures 5.8a and 5.8b

SPACING ISSUES

Spacing issues are usually corrected after all of the adult teeth have come into the mouth. However, excess spacing on the upper front teeth is often correlated with impacted upper adult canine teeth, as shown in the following panoramic x-ray (see Figure 5.9). If this condition is identified early enough, your orthodontist may recommend the removal of the baby canines. When the upper adult canines are poorly positioned, as they are on the above x-ray, and the baby canines are removed early enough, research has shown that the upper adult canines have about a 60 percent chance of coming into the mouth. When the upper adult canines are poorly positioned and the baby canines are not removed, there is virtually a 100 percent chance that the upper adult canines will become impacted and will require a surgery to bring them into the mouth. In some cases, upper adult impacted canines can damage the roots of the adult upper incisors and cause them to be lost in early adulthood.[20] It is, therefore, imperative that poorly positioned upper adult canines be identified and addressed as early as possible.

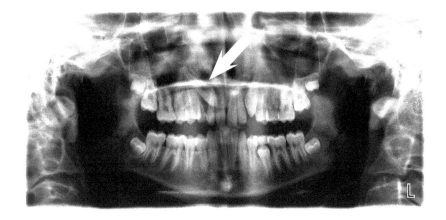

Figure 5.9

I can't emphasize enough the importance of taking your child for an orthodontic evaluation by age seven, like the AAO advises. Your child may not need braces right away, but it may be important to remove some baby teeth in the case of spacing issues, or just to evaluate for gum recession in the case of an crossbite. Early evaluation may require a phase 1 treatment, but the overall treatment plan would be much less invasive for your child and that would be a good thing. However, if you are an adult and you have an issue like a severe underbite or an open bite issue that should have been addressed earlier, do not lose hope. As I said previously, I have never encountered a problem I could not treat and I can assure you there

---

20   Susan M. Power and Mary B. E. Short, "An Investigation into the Response of Palatally Displaced Canines to the Removal of Deciduous Canines and an Assessment of Factors Contributing to Favourable Eruption," *British Journal of Orthodontics* 20, no. 3 (1993): 215–223, https://doi.org/10.1179/bjo.20.3.215; John H. Warford Jr. et al., "Prediction of maxillary canine impaction using sectors and angular measurement," *American Journal of Orthodontics & Dentofacial Orthopedics* 124, no. 6 (2003): 651–655, https://doi.org/10.1016/S0889-5406(03)00621-8

is a highly-qualified orthodontist in your area that could make the same claim. Sometimes the treatment is more extensive, takes longer, and may even require surgical intervention, but the end result can always be a healthy, beautiful smile.

—DR. VERBIC

chapter six

EXPANDERS: WHAT THEY ARE AND WHEN THEY ARE USED

Expanders—just the name sounds a bit frightening. You can assume from the name that expanders are used to expand something, but what exactly do they expand in the mouth, why is expansion sometimes necessary and wouldn't expanding something in the mouth be painful?

Many orthodontists use these devices to treat crossbites, crowding, and impacted teeth. There is another reason expanders are sometimes used—breathing problems—but this is quite controversial (we will talk about it a bit later). Expanders can be used on the upper and lower teeth. When used on the upper teeth, they are called "palatal expanders" because they work to stretch (or widen) the bone of the upper dental palate to make more room for the teeth and to move teeth within the jaw. When used on the lower teeth, they only work to move the teeth; use of lower expanders is less common.

HOW EXPANDERS WORK

There are many different types of expanders but they all look similar and work in the same way. Figure 6.1 shows an example of what an expander looks like placed on the upper teeth. I know it looks a bit strange, maybe even scary or painful, but it doesn't hurt to place it on the teeth, and most patients only experience minor discomfort for a short period of time after every adjustment or turning of the expander.

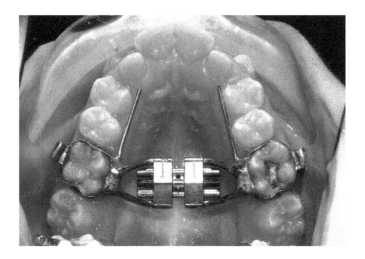

Figure 6.1

An expander is typically placed with an intermediate-strength adhesive so it will not come off of the teeth at an inopportune time. This will allow it to be removed easily when it is no longer needed. Placement of an expander usually requires one visit to size up the bands that hold the expander on the teeth and one visit to bond the expander to the teeth. At both the band-sizing visit and the bonding visit, pressure is applied to the bands to fit them snuggly around the teeth. This snug fit also prevents the expander from coming off the teeth on its own. The pressure is applied by having the patient bite down on a plastic stick to push the bands over the teeth. The glue that is used to bond the expander to the teeth usually contains fluoride to prevent any cavities from forming underneath the bands.

For expanders to function properly, the keyhole in the middle must be turned by the patient or a parent. Your orthodontist should tell you how often to turn the expander key and how often he or she would like to check on the progress of the expansion so the desired result may be achieved. Your orthodontist should also show you how to turn the key and make sure you are able to do so on your own. Depending on how often your orthodontist tells you to turn the key, the period of actively turning an expander usually lasts one to twelve weeks. Expanders are usually left in place for several more months after the turning is done so that the resulting expansion does not relapse.

GOOD AND BAD CANDIDATES FOR EXPANDERS

Expanders are used frequently by many orthodontists today. An orthodontist may prescribe an expander to correct a posterior crossbite or to gain space when teeth are crowded. They are used more often in younger patients than in older patients because they are more effective at an earlier age. The sutures of the palate do not fuse until puberty, which is why expanders are most effective prior to the age of thirteen or fourteen years old. In these children, expanders lead to very predictable results. Crossbite correction is very stable and much room can be gained for children with crowded teeth.

When expanders are used after the sutures fuse, they will either be ineffective or will lead to an unstable result. This means crossbites that are corrected after puberty with an expander will typically relapse. For adults who have posterior crossbites, a surgical procedure may be required to reopen the sutures prior to the use of an expander. Alternatively, adults with posterior crossbites may choose to accept a less-than-ideal result by foregoing the use of an expander and not correcting the crossbite. However, if a crossbite in an adult is mild, it may still be corrected with an expander. This correction will likely be due to tipping of the upper back teeth and not from an expansion of the sutures. Tipping of the back teeth is not usually stable, however, and long-term retainer wear will be required to prevent the crossbite from returning.

Parents who had expanders when they were young are typically less concerned about them being prescribed for their own children because they are familiar with them. But when parents are unfamiliar with them, use of expanders in their children can lead to anxiety on the part of both the parent and child. If your orthodontist does prescribe an expander, he or she should take the time to show you and your child what one looks like, how it is placed, approximately how long it will remain on the teeth, how it is removed, and what to expect in terms of eating and speaking.

CONTROVERSIAL USE OF EXPANDERS

Previously, I mentioned a controversial use of expanders to address breathing problems in children. Breathing problems in children are serious. In fact, a lack of oxygen intake can lead to symptoms resembling ADHD in children, failure to thrive, and an inability to concentrate in school. It is thought that 50 percent of children diagnosed with ADHD may simply not be getting enough oxygen due to a restricted air intake.[21] Sometimes, dentists and orthodontists recommend the use of an expander to address these breathing problems in a child. The idea is that the expander will increase the

---

21   Stefan Baumgartner and Martina Eichenberger, "The Impact of Rapid Palatal Expansion on Children's General Health: A Literature Review," *Journal of Paediatric Dentistry* 15, no. 1 (March 2014): 67–71, https://doi.org/10.5167/uzh-94158

volume of air these children take in when breathing as a result of the widening of the upper palate. There is no doubt expanders do increase the volume of the nasal cavity, but so far there is not enough evidence this increase significantly improves breathing in children, or that it can lead to better overall health outcomes. If your child is snoring at night or habitually breathes through their mouth, it is important to have an evaluation by an Ear, Nose, and Throat physician. Common causes of snoring and mouth breathing include obesity, allergies, and enlarged tonsils and adenoids. Both allergies and enlarged tonsils and adenoids can adversely affect the growth of the jaws and may cause posterior crossbites. Yes, expanders can be used to fix the crossbites. However, addressing the obesity, allergies, or enlarged tonsils and adenoids are proven means to help children breathe better. The use of expanders is not. Beware of any orthodontist who tells you that this is a good reason to use an expander.

MINOR ISSUES (ANNOYANCES, REALLY) WITH EXPANDERS

Children usually experience mild soreness after an expander is turned each time.[22] This soreness tends to last fewer than fifteen minutes. It is unusual to need pain medication, but an over-the-counter pain reliever, such as acetaminophen or Ibuprofen can be taken thirty minutes prior to turning the expander, if needed.

The most frequently reported issue with expanders is the fact that children have difficulty getting used to eating with them in place.[23] Swallowing can become more difficult because the tongue can no longer touch the palate with the expander in place and chewing may feel and be different for your child. However, children usually adjust

---

22   Cheryl Zaidan, "How to Live with a Palate Expander," Oral Health, HealDove, https://healdove.com/oral-health/palateexpander

23   Ibid.

to eating within twenty-four hours of getting the expander. Just after getting the expander, it is probably a good idea for your child to eat liquid foods, such as Jell-O or soups. As your child adapts to eating with the expander, it is ok to add soft solid foods at first and then a normal diet. It is always a good idea for your child to cut larger or tougher pieces of food (such as meat) into smaller bites throughout the duration of treatment with the expander.

Another issue with the placement of an expander is excessive saliva. This can cause a lot of drooling, especially while your child is sleeping and the jaw is relaxed. Speech issues can also be a concern. Having an expander on the roof of the mouth causes the tongue to be positioned differently and can cause your child to have a lisp and experience difficulty pronouncing words, specifically words that start with S, G, X, or Z. It may take a while for your child to get used to formulating words and sounds using his or her tongue around the expander, but speech sounds should improve over time.

The good news is that all the issues discussed above are generally short lived and should go away after several weeks.

WHY I RARELY USE EXPANDERS

Not all orthodontists use expanders or feel they are always necessary to correct crossbites and crowded teeth. In my own experience, and in the experience of other orthodontists, the same results can be achieved by braces alone. There are rare cases of severe, bilateral cross-bites where the use of an expander is necessary, but in the majority of cases, braces alone can expand the upper teeth out of a crossbite.

Parents and children who are anxious or afraid of wearing an expander are, needless to say, often relieved to find out they don't need an expander. Still, some parents insist their orthodontist use an expander because that's what worked for their crowding or crossbite when they were a child. The decision to include an expander in treatment should be discussed by the parent, patient and orthodontist on a case-by-case basis.

> *Expanders do work and many orthodontists rely on them as a gold standard, but after learning how to use them effectively and using them in the early days of my practice with success, I now use them rarely, if at all, and here is why: I had been hearing for years about orthodontists who stopped using them. I thought these orthodontists were avant garde, and I knew intuitively that it was possible to treat most orthodontic issues with braces alone to avoid the use of expanders, but I didn't consider limiting my use of them because I hadn't personally met an orthodontist who wasn't using them. Then, I met an orthodontist with a practice forty minutes south of me who had stopped using them more than a decade ago and was running a very successful orthodontic practice. He was doing a really good job on peoples' teeth; I saw his finished product in several of his patients. I thought to myself that if he can do this and his patient's teeth look so good, then I certainly can do this. So, I stopped using them and it is much, much easier on my patients. But, it's almost heresy to say I don't use them in our community, because 99 percent of orthodontists do."*

> **—DR. VERBIC**

It's a really good idea to get a second opinion before agreeing to treatment with an expander for your child for any reason because most orthodontic issues can be addressed with braces alone. There are very limited reasons for the use of an expander as an essential part of treatment.

BRACES ARE NOT WHAT THEY USED TO BE

Can you believe it has taken us until chapter seven to discuss braces? I guess there is just so much to talk about regarding the decision making of starting orthodontic treatment that the actual discussion of braces becomes a bit of an afterthought. Really, once the decision is made to proceed with orthodontic treatment, the treatment devices themselves are not hugely important or even interesting to many people. However, this is a shame because it's fascinating how braces work … at least to me.

At each of my patients' initial exams, I ask them, no matter how young or old they are, how and what they have thought about being treated. Most haven't given it too much thought; they are really focused more on the outcome, not the process. This is great, but I always try to explain a bit about the process so they are 100 percent invested in their treatment plan (which, as I have discussed, is key to faster treatment times). I usually discuss the type of braces I will be using and give a brief talk about the steps of treatment, including how long treatment will last, and answer any questions patients might have. So, I will begin here with a discussion about the different parts that make up the braces and the types of braces and brackets that are available.

COMPONENTS OF BRACES

There are basically two types of braces available today: conventional (or traditional) and self-ligating. We will discuss the differences between the two types a bit later. Both of these braces use brackets, bonding material, and arch wires. Conventional braces also use ligature elastics to hold each bracket onto the arch wire.

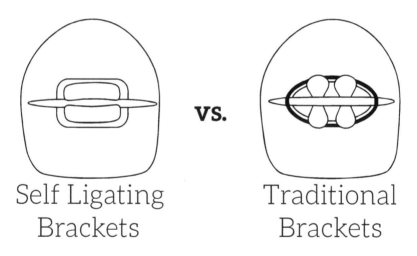

Figure 7.1

Brackets are made of either metal or ceramic.[24] Most patients use metal brackets, but a growing number are choosing ceramic brackets because they are far less noticeable on the teeth (we will talk about this a little later, too). Brackets are attached or bonded onto each tooth in the mouth by use of a sealant and a glue-like substance, none of which will harm the enamel of the teeth. After each bracket is placed, an arch wire, which is a thin metal wire that attaches to each bracket and is placed bracket to bracket, is placed. It is the arch wire that, when tightened, puts pressure on the teeth to move them. The ligature elastic (sometimes called the O-ring) is used in conventional braces to attach the arch wire to the bracket. In self-ligating brackets, the arch wire connects directly to the bracket using a metal clip or gate (Figure 7.2).

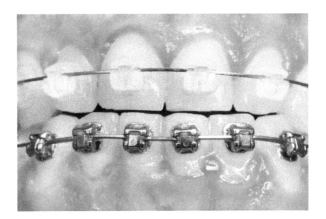

Figure 7.2

24 "How Do Braces Work? A Basic Explanation," Archwired, www.archwired. com/how_braces_work.htm; Eric Leber, "Bonding Braces to Your Teeth," Leber Ortho, http://leberortho.com/patient-info/braces-blog/bonding-braces-to-your-teeth; "5-Star-Rated Orthodontist for Damon Braces in Palantine & Barrington, IL," Verbic Orthodontics, https://palatinebraces.com/braces-and-invisalign-palatine-barrington-illinois-il/damon-braces/

TYPES OF BRACES AND BRACKETS

So, what is the difference between conventional braces and self-ligating braces? The difference is just in the way the arch wire connects to the bracket, as discussed above. Both types of braces are extremely effective in treatment outcomes. However, self-ligating braces are a much newer technology, and thus, there are, in my opinion, significant improvements in design and improvements in speed of treatment. Because self-ligating braces use a gate to attach the bracket to the arch wire, the system is more door-like. The use of metal clips or gates instead of elastics allows for a more constant, light force on the teeth compared to conventional braces because in conventional braces, the rubber ties lose their elasticity every few days, whereas the gates on the self-ligating braces do not. In addition, this new style of braces is sleeker, which results in a more streamlined look. Patients enjoy the same level of comfort as with traditional braces. Also, because the rubber ties are not needed to attach the bracket to the arch wire, there is less chance for food particles to be trapped, leading to decreased risk for cavities and gum disease. Self-ligating braces also require less-frequent visits to the orthodontist for tightening. Traditional braces require a visit about every four weeks, while self-ligating braces require a visit only about every eight to ten weeks. Finally, another advantage of this newer technology is reduced treatment time due to the fact that with self-ligating braces, there is a more constant, light force on the teeth.

In addition to the types of braces systems, there are also different types of brackets available—metal (stainless steel or titanium), ceramic, or plastic. There are pros and cons to each type, depending on each individual patient, and the choice is usually made after a discussion with the orthodontist. I do have an interesting brackets story to tell you about a patient of mine, though. Most of my patients have no issues using metal brackets, but there are some people who have an allergy to metal and they usually do not even know it.

> *One of my patients had metal braces placed and, within a week, her lips and gums were very swollen. Turns out she had an allergy to the stainless-steel metal used in the braces. A switch to titanium metal braces for this patient fixed the problem. This type of reaction is not normal. So, if you know you have an allergy to stainless steel or nickel, or you experience severe swelling in your lips or gums after you get your braces, please inform your orthodontist. The use of titanium or ceramic braces will alleviate the discomfort and create a more pleasant experience throughout your treatment.*
>
> **—DR. VERBIC**

We have talked about the components of braces and types of braces systems and brackets, but not really about how braces work. In the general discussion of braces with each of my patients, I don't usually discuss how braces *actually* work to straighten teeth because not every patient cares very much. Only about 10 percent of my patients are interested in *how* braces straighten the teeth. For those 10 percent, I love to get into the details. So, briefly, for the 10 per-centers out there, here goes.

HOW BRACES WORK TO STRAIGHTEN TEETH

As I said previously, the arch wire is what puts pressure on the teeth, causing them to move. In addition, elastics are sometimes placed on the brackets connecting the top teeth with the bottom teeth.[25] These elastics apply additional pressure and are used to help move not only the position of the teeth, but also the position of the jaws to correct a patient's misaligned bite. All this pressure, over time, causes the

---

25   "How Do Braces Work?" Archwired, www.archwired.com/how_braces_work.htm

teeth to move in the direction intended by the orthodontist. It is the orthodontist who positions the brackets, arch wires and, if necessary, elastics in such a way as to exert pressure in the correct manner and position, which allows the teeth to move in the proper direction.

How the teeth move is caused by a process called bone remodeling. Although this sounds very technical, it is such a cool biomechanical process. Basically, when pressure is applied to the teeth, the teeth loosen within the gums, periodontal ligaments and the bone in which the teeth sit (it is called the alveolar bone) (see Figure 7.3). This process stimulates the alveolar bone to remodel.

The exciting thing about bone is that it breaks down, regenerates, grows, and strengthens when stimulated. When force is applied to bone, cells called osteoclasts rush in to break down the bone. However, it doesn't stop there. When the force is removed, cells called osteoblasts rush to the site to build new bone. When this process is repeated over time, the bone density increases.

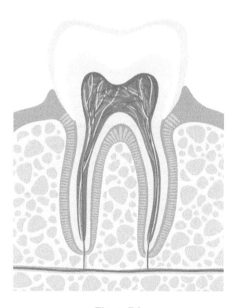

Figure 7.3

With the teeth and braces, it works like this—when the alveolar bone is stimulated by the applied force (braces), osteoclasts move to the site to break down the bone, allowing the teeth to loosen and move in the desired direction. Then, osteoblasts take over and begin to build new bone around the new position of the teeth. Over many months, this process of repeated breaking down of the bone (stimulation caused by pressure exerted on the teeth) leads to movement of teeth and repair of bone around the new positioning. The end result is perfect positioning of teeth in strong alveolar bone, which is necessary for keeping your new beautiful smile in place. The process takes time, which is why I always tell patients that the estimated time in braces is twenty-two months. Of course, the process can occur faster in some people and slower in others, depending a lot on the factors we discussed in previous chapters.

There it is. A very cool process, no? Now you know everything there is to know about braces and how they work. You will be the most educated orthodontic patient (or parent of a patient) ever.

Braces are really amazing. They were, and still are, a great invention; they have revolutionized aesthetic dental care and changed the lives of so many people. Their design continues to develop and improve and they are, and will remain, a standard of orthodontic care for years to come. But—and you just knew there was a but coming—there is a relatively new tool in the orthodontist's toolkit that is even more amazing (if that's even possible).

chapter eight

THE INCREDIBLE INVENTION
OF INVISALIGN

The relatively new tool in the orthodontist's toolkit are clear aligners, the most popular being the product Invisalign. In the last fifteen years, nothing has revolutionized orthodontic treatment quite like Invisalign has. Invisalign is a custom-made series of clear aligners that straighten teeth without the patient having to wear braces. That's right, no metal brackets and arch wires; instead, clear aligner trays that can be removed for eating, drinking, and dental hygiene. Figure 8.1 shows what an Invisalign tray looks like off of the teeth.

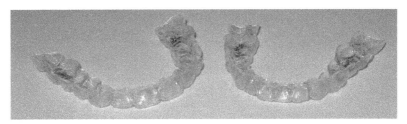

Figure 8.1

There is great interest in Invisalign. Just saying this is really an understatement. Over the past several years, as this technology became more well-known and well respected, the majority of my new patients would bring it up to me by asking whether or not they would be good candidates for this treatment. Now, I bring up Invisalign with each new patient in every single exam, whether or not I go on to recommend this treatment for the particular patient. For those who are not candidates for Invisalign, it's important for them to know why, because many people want to use this technology and are disappointed when they can't for whatever reason. Invisalign is very popular and has caused a boom in orthodontic treatment, especially among adults.

—DR. VERBIC

CREATING YOUR PERSONALIZED INVISALIGN TRAYS

If you and your orthodontist decide Invisalign is right for you, your orthodontist will take a digital impression of your teeth with a scanner or with traditional impression trays. These impressions will be sent to Invisalign and the technicians at the company will create a virtual treatment simulation called a ClinCheck. Your orthodontist will interact with Invisalign's technicians using the ClinCheck to virtually construct the sequence of aligners that will move your teeth to their correct positions. When your orthodontist is comfortable with the virtual sequence of aligners, he or she will approve it and the technicians will construct your personalized Invisalign aligner trays from a proprietary plastic via 3-D printing. It generally takes three to six weeks for this process to take place and for the aligners to be shipped to your orthodontist's office.

HOW INVISALIGN WORKS

Before you start treatment with your aligner trays, your orthodontist must bond Invisalign attachments to your teeth. The attachments on your teeth are made out of the same clear adhesive that is used to bond braces to teeth, and they are placed in a similar manner to braces. They can be irritating to the cheeks and lips when the aligners are not in the mouth but patients quickly adapt to them. I find that most patients adapt to these attachments much easier and much more quickly than is the case with traditional braces. The aligner trays push and pull on the attachments bonded to your teeth in order to move your teeth. Without these attachments, the movements the aligner trays are capable of would be severely limited. In fact, the attachments are a major reason why orthodontic treatment with Invisalign has become so mainstream. Between the years 2000 and 2005, the design of the attachments was rudimentary and the number of people that could be treated with Invisalign was quite limited. Treatment was also less predictable than it is today. Many orthodontists gave up on using Invisalign during this time because of poor results. Since 2005, the engineers at Invisalign have continued to improve upon the attachments, and both the movement of teeth and the results of treatment have become much more predictable. Your orthodontist determines the design of the attachments, and which teeth they are placed on to achieve the desired movements of your teeth. The tooth movement is achieved in the exact same way as was discussed in chapter seven. The aligners exert force/pressure on the teeth, causing the process of bone breakdown, tooth movement and bone regrowth (bone remodeling) … all without the use of brackets or arch wires. Pretty cool.

ADVANTAGES OF INVISALIGN

From the patient's perspective, the main advantage of Invisalign over braces is that Invisalign is virtually invisible and undetectable to most people, even at a conversational distance (Figure 8.2). Another advantage is that the trays are removable so it is possible for patients to eat the foods they would normally eat without fear of breaking braces off of their teeth. In addition, the fact that the trays are removable also mean it's easy for patients to keep their teeth clean by brushing and flossing. Patients who wear braces must spend considerably more time and effort to brush and floss compared to patients who wear Invisalign. When patients do not invest enough time and effort in their oral hygiene while wearing braces, it can lead to a characteristic pattern of decalcification and decay. Typically, patients who are undergoing treatment with Invisalign will also have less frequent visits to their orthodontist for adjustments than they would with braces. Braces require adjustments every two to ten weeks, whereas adjustments with Invisalign occur every eight to fourteen weeks, or even longer.

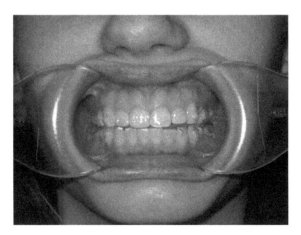

Figure 8.2

A good portion of my patients are being treated with Invisalign. Some of these patients have never worn braces, but others may have had braces as a child or teenager, and for reasons listed previously in the book, needed additional treatment. Generally speaking, the patients who had braces when they were younger and are now being treated with Invisalign *love* Invisalign and say it is the best thing ever. Those patients who never had braces or any other type of orthodontic treatment are not quite as thrilled.

Remember Susan, my patient who had braces as a teenager, hated them and then years later came to see me in hopes of re-straightening her teeth? She is one of my patients who loved Invisalign in comparison to braces. She really liked the appearance, freedom, and comfort of Invisalign. She loved how no one could tell she had the trays in, and she loved that she could take them out to eat and brush her teeth. She loved their comfort compared to the old-fashioned metal braces she had had as a teenager. For her, it was a great experience and, because of this, she wore her trays as instructed and finished treatment on time. I have treated many patients like Susan and they are so happy with Invisalign. I have also treated many patients whose first experience with orthodontic treatment was Invisalign. One of my patients in this category was a twenty-one-year-old college student. He would complain to me on occasion that having to wear the aligner trays twenty-two hours out of the day was sometimes really difficult. He liked to eat out and go to the bar with his friends and he found it difficult to adhere to the twenty-two hours per day recommended time to wear the aligners. But, he told me he wouldn't complain too much because his mom kept telling him how much better he had it compared to the braces she had to wear for two years when she was a teenager.

—DR. VERBIC

KEY POINTS ON CHOOSING INVISALIGN

The main concern orthodontists have when treating patients with Invisalign is that the Invisalign trays are removable which, as you just read, is one of the key reasons patients love Invisalign. Invisalign works the same way that braces work: by applying a light, but *constant,* force to the teeth. When the aligners are not being worn, they cannot apply this force. Thus, for optimal results, Invisalign recommends the patient wear the Invisalign aligners for at least twenty-two hours a day. Yes, twenty-two out of the twenty-four hours in a day!

In my experience, when the aligners are not worn for at least eighteen hours a day, nothing is being accomplished. This is because during the time the aligners are not being worn, the teeth are rebounding to their previous positions. When patients do not faithfully wear their aligners for at least twenty-two hours per day, additional aligners must be ordered to achieve the desired result. This can add many months on to the treatment length, many additional visits to the orthodontist's office and increased costs. The best approach is to plan to wear your aligners for at least twenty-two hours per day, but to understand that most patients cannot adhere to this amount of wear and to not be disappointed if you need to have additional aligners ordered to achieve your desired result.

This concern about Invisalign is the advantage that treatment with braces has, especially from the orthodontist's perspective. With braces, patients do not have a choice to remove anything because the braces cannot be removed by the patient. As a parent, this may be something to consider if your teen is a candidate for Invisalign. Some teenagers are mature and disciplined enough to adhere to wearing (and not losing) the Invisalign aligner trays; some are not. Only you know your child.

The other concern with choosing Invisalign over braces is that Invisalign, by itself, cannot correct your bite. This may or may not be important to you (see chapter three). A patient's bite can be corrected the same way it can be with traditional braces—by using orthodontic elastics. However, these elastics are noticeable when they are being worn with Invisalign. This effectively negates one of the appeals of Invisalign—the fact that it's invisible. It is best to discuss what bothers you about your smile or your bite with your orthodontist. If your bite does not feel comfortable or you have a large overbite or underbite you feel is unsightly, then it may be better to choose treatment with braces rather than with Invisalign.

Finally, Invisalign is not for everyone. If it was, you probably wouldn't see as many people still wearing braces. Certain tooth movements (rotations, intrusions, extrusions, and tipping) are too severe for Invisalign alone to correct in an efficient and timely manner. Also, some people choose braces over Invisalign because they do not think they will be good about keeping the aligners on their teeth for twenty-two hours or more a day, every day for a year. Other people feel like they will misplace aligners. And others, especially children, want to wear the variety of colors that come with traditional braces.

Together with your orthodontist, you can choose the treatment modality that is right for you and/or your child.

chapter nine

DON'T BE SCARED: THE TRUTH ABOUT PAIN AND TREATMENT

One of the biggest fears in going to the orthodontist is, "Is this going to hurt? That expander looks huge! Will it hurt the inside of my mouth? Does it hurt to put the braces on? Does it hurt to wear them? Does it hurt to take them off?" Even, "Does Invisalign hurt?" My practice has surveyed thousands of patients over the years to rate their pain on a scale of one to ten. The results come back with an average of three out of ten. Most patients experience the most discomfort from the teeth moving within one to four days of first getting their expander, braces, or Invisalign. So that first week of treatment is really the biggest adjustment, usually because the experience is brand new to most people. During these first few days, orthodontists recommend eating softer foods, like soups and yogurts. They also recommend not eating tougher foods, like whole apples, or chewing on really hard, sticky things, such as Tootsie rolls or beef jerky, or any foods that are going to make your teeth sore. If needed, a mild pain reliever, such as over-the-counter acetaminophen or ibuprofen, may be taken. After approximately the first week of wearing your expander, braces, or Invisalign trays, things return to normal for the duration of treatment and harder foods usually do not cause any discomfort.

RELIEVING FEAR AND ANXIETY

While there is some minor pain and discomfort associated with orthodontic treatment, fear and anxiety are the bigger culprits in hindering patients, especially at the beginning of treatment. This is why I believe addressing these factors is just as important as providing tips on dealing with pain and discomfort. My head orthodontic assistant is instrumental in putting our patients at ease when they walk into our office. So, I'll let you read what she has to say about this topic of fear and anxiety.

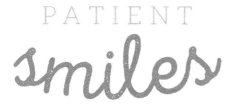

One of several patients I've seen was incredibly nervous when she started treatment. For the past year, she's been transformed into a totally different patient when she visits for her appointments. I was reflecting on this and decided to ask her what it was that made her change. I asked her, "What was it that put you at ease?"

She said, "I just got to know all of you; you are all just people."

It hit me; building a relationship with each patient is key. It is so important for all of us in our office to build a personal relationship with each of our patients because this is one of the most important things that makes them feel comfortable. And when patients are comfortable, then fear, anxiety, and even pain are lessened.

It's all about the read on the patient. In the initial relationship, I want each of my patients to know I am hearing them, and that I understand they are nervous and will work with them to meet their needs and make them feel comfortable. Sometimes, making them feel comfortable takes time and we get a bit behind in treatment. This is ok; once they feel comfortable, we can catch up with the treatment.

We treated a patient in her fifties who was initially one of the most anxious patients we had ever met. So, we adapted her treatment to what she could handle at each visit. For example, we said, "Let's change one wire today and then make another appointment to change the other wire. Just because we are supposed to put two wires in doesn't mean we have to do it today." We also asked her, "Are you ready?" before proceeding with any treatment. We gave the control back to her so she felt like she could own her treatment. Guess what? This same patient now falls asleep in the chair at every appointment!

Another patient began treatment when she was very young. She was so nervous and scared at her first appointment, it took almost an hour to put rubber band separators in between her teeth. She kept telling us to wait, wait, wait. A year later, she can hardly believe she was that patient. She still wants every new step in her treatment explained to her, but she is relaxed and we are very happy to explain everything.

We always make sure to tell our patients that they can always ask questions. Even if they don't ask questions, we always explain everything to them. We would never throw a treatment technique at a patient without an explanation. Communication is key. We also always talk to parents of younger patients after each appointment. We tell parents what happened during the appointment and what will happen at the next appointment.

Building a relationship, making sure the patient feels comfortable and at ease and ensuring good communication are key to alleviating fear and anxiety, which, in turn, really does lessen pain and discomfort. But, of course, there is a physical aspect too. When helping patients deal with physical pain and discomfort, it is important for us to realize that every one of our patients is different and that everyone's pain tolerance is different.

One pain-relieving technique might not work for every patient. And, it is up to us to find what works best for each of our patients. That said, the information provided below by Dr. Verbic are the pain- and discomfort-relieving techniques that work the best for the patients we have seen in our office. —MEGAN M., HEAD ORTHODONTIC ASSISTANT AT VERBIC ORTHODONTICS

RELIEVING THE DISCOMFORT ASSOCIATED WITH EXPANDERS

We talked a bit about the pain associated with expanders in chapter six. Since the expander is working to actually move or widen the upper palate, there is going to be some soreness associated with this process. Generally, there is some initial soreness or discomfort after first getting an expander, and with each adjustment or turning of the key. However, the discomfort is usually mild and can be controlled with over-the-counter acetaminophen or ibuprofen.

In addition to soreness, you may experience some swelling. Taking over-the-counter ibuprofen will definitely help with any swelling, and you can also use a hot compress or washcloth on the site where it is painful for up to ten minutes at a time.

RELIEVING THE DISCOMFORT ASSOCIATED WITH BRACES

When an orthodontist is placing the braces on your teeth, you will not feel any pain at all. In fact, many patients fall asleep in the chair because it can sometimes take up to an hour to complete the process. The orthodontist and their assistants prepare the teeth so a bonding resin or glue will adhere to them. It is this bonding resin that makes it possible to simply stick the braces to the teeth, whether the braces are made out of stainless steel, titanium, or ceramic. Gone are the days when orthodontists needed to push and pry bands around every single tooth. This antiquated procedure was quite uncomfortable and when bonding resins came into the market, they made a drastic improvement in patient comfort. The preparation of teeth for bonding the brackets and the adhesive resin can taste bad during the procedure, but an orthodontist and assistant can minimize this bad taste by being careful to keep the materials away from the taste buds on the tongue. In any case, the materials used by orthodontists to both prepare the teeth and to adhere the braces to the teeth are non-toxic, even if they have a bad taste.

During the time patients wear braces, the lips and cheeks (and, in the case of lingual braces, especially the tongue) can become irritated by the braces. Most patients adjust to this irritation within the first week of treatment. I like to compare it to building up calluses on your fingers when playing the guitar. After your lips and cheeks adapt, they will no longer be sore or irritated from the braces. The orthodontist will give you an inert wax that can be applied to the braces in the areas causing irritation for relief until the cheeks and lips can adapt. Rarely, the braces can contribute to an increase in canker sores in the mouth. Researchers aren't sure what causes canker sores, but braces can increase their occurrence. Fortunately, there are many over-the-counter remedies for canker sores. For immediate and complete pain relief, your dentist or orthodontist can provide treatment with Debacterol.

It is rare that patients make it through treatment with braces without a pokey wire. The poke usually occurs on the part of the cheek close to the top, back teeth. The wires responsible for straightening the teeth can sometime move out of the back either accidentally, through the normal process of chewing food, or as an unavoidable part of treatment, like closing gaps between teeth. The same wax used at the start of treatment can be used for temporary relief until you are able to return to the orthodontist to have the wire trimmed.

If the pokey wire is very uncomfortable and you cannot return to the orthodontist soon to have it trimmed, you may attempt to do so yourself with a pair of fingernail clippers. Be very careful, though, as fingernail clippers are very sharp and may cut any part of the mouth. Alternatively, you can attempt to push the wire back into place with the eraser end of a pencil.

Most patients experience mild to no discomfort when braces are removed. Many patients are so excited to see their new smile for the first time they are not even thinking of what it is like to have the braces removed. Some patients, however, do feel mild discomfort upon removal of the braces. This is more prevalent in patients who have not maintained good oral hygiene habits during their treatment because of inflammation in the gums and in the periodontal ligament that holds the teeth in the jaws. If you have experienced some discomfort during adjustment or "tightening" appointments, it may be a good idea to take over-the-counter acetaminophen or ibuprofen thirty minutes prior to removal of the braces. After the braces are removed, the adhesive resin used to stick the braces to the teeth is polished off. The reason why the adhesive does not come off when the braces are taken of the teeth is that the adhesive is designed to break from the braces before it breaks from the teeth. If it was designed to break from the teeth first and come off with the braces, the enamel could be permanently damaged. (As a side note, the first ceramic brackets that came out on the market approximately thirty years ago, unfortunately, caused this exact problem. Fortunately, the braces manufacturers redesigned them to solve this problem.)

The orthodontist uses a polishing device that looks a lot like the hand piece that a dentist uses to perform fillings, and this can understandably make patients quite nervous. But not to fear, the device the orthodontist uses to polish the adhesive from the teeth does not damage the tooth in any way. A minority of patients can experience "cold chills" in their teeth during the polishing procedure. This can be due to the vibration of the polishing device or from the "cold" air that device uses to operate. Patients with gum recession are more susceptible to discomfort during adhesive removal because the roots of their teeth are exposed to the cold air from the polishing device. If you have had discomfort during cleanings at the dentist from the cold water that is used, you may experience similar discomfort with adhesive removal. If this is the case, it is probably a good idea to take over-the-counter acetaminophen or ibuprofen thirty minutes prior to your appointment for braces removal. In any case, the anesthesia that a dentist uses to "numb up" patients prior to dental procedures is never required. And that means you'll never need a shot at the orthodontist's office.

RELIEVING THE DISCOMFORT ASSOCIATED WITH INVISALIGN

The experience with Invisalign is similar to braces. The attachments placed to help the aligners move the teeth are placed using the same methods and materials that the orthodontist uses with braces. These attachments can also irritate the lips and cheeks, just as braces do. Wax is usually not needed, however, as simply having the aligners in place will provide relief. The discomfort that patients experience for the first few days with braces is also same for patients with their first set of Invisalign aligners and should subside within a few days. When subsequent aligners are placed, there can be a milder discomfort that is usually shorter in duration than the first set of Invisalign aligners. During treatment, one of the advantages of Invisalign over braces is that there are no wires needed to straighten your teeth. That means there is no possibility of pokey wires or the extra trip to the orthodontist office to have them trimmed.

Invisalign attachments are also removed with the same polishing device that is used to remove adhesive resin from the teeth after a patient has worn braces. The experience of having attachments removed is very much the same as having adhesive resin from braces removed. A word of caution, though . . . never have your attachments removed within one week of whitening or bleaching your teeth. Ask me how I know? The whitening agents can cause extreme sensitivity in the teeth and make the attachment removal process impossible without a numbing shot of anesthetic.

The key sentence in this chapter is, "You'll never need a shot at the orthodontist's office." Yes, there is minor pain and discomfort associated with orthodontic treatment, but as you have read, it is easily handled. It is very important to find and choose an orthodontic practice where you feel very comfortable and at ease, where all your questions are respected and answered and where your fears and anxieties are taken seriously.

chapter ten

THE DREADED TOOTH EXTRACTION: FACTS ABOUT PERMANENT TOOTH REMOVAL

Most people can look at their teeth in the mirror and see whether their teeth are crowded. But the question that people with crowded teeth often ask is, "Am I going have to have teeth taken out to make enough room to straighten out my smile?" This was often the case twenty to twenty-five years ago. Back then, by some estimates, 76 percent of patients had teeth removed as part of their orthodontic treatment.[26] Since those times, however, braces and treatment methodologies have advanced, and today, extractions of adult teeth can usually be avoided. We will get back to this point later in the chapter.

---

26 William R. Proffit, "Forty-year review of extraction frequencies at a university orthodontic clinic," *The Angle Orthodontist* 64, no. 6 (1994): 407–414, https://www.ncbi.nlm.nih.gov/pubmed/7864461

One of the main reasons orthodontists advocate that children have an exam by the age of seven is to determine whether children are at risk for severe crowding once all of the adult teeth have erupted. If they are, then the orthodontist can provide treatment to the child before all of the adult teeth have erupted. Treatment involves creating enough room in the mouth for all the teeth so that, in the great majority of cases, extractions can be avoided. This is usually accomplished with braces, space maintainers, and/or expanders.

The more-difficult scenario occurs after all of the adult teeth have erupted into the mouth. At this point, the ability to make enough room for all of the teeth in a severely crowded situation is much more limited, but it can be done. Frankly, most orthodontists will readily admit that no matter how severely crowded a patient's teeth are, they can always be straightened with braces or Invisalign. But this misses the point, for a few specific reasons.

REASONS WHY ADULT TOOTH REMOVAL MAY BE NECESSARY IN CASES OF SEVERE CROWDING

Using braces or Invisalign to straighten severely crowded teeth misses the point, because when severely crowded teeth are simply straightened, the health of some of the teeth (usually the front teeth) may be jeopardized. This is because as the teeth are being aligned, they can be pushed out of the bone holding them in the jaws. When this happens, unsightly gum recession and even loosening of the teeth may occur. Figure 10.1 provides an example of gum recession after straightening of severely crowded teeth.

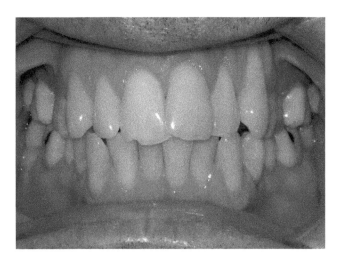

Figure 10.1

PREVENTING GUM RECESSION

In order to prevent this from occurring, your orthodontist should perform a thorough initial exam to determine treatment options and to give you a prediction of whether recession will occur during alignment of your teeth. If your orthodontist thinks recession is a strong possibility, then tooth removal should be recommended.

PREVENTING A PROTRUSIVE SMILE

In addition to the possibility of gum recession occurring, simply straightening teeth in patients with severe crowding of teeth may also lead to what orthodontists call a "protrusive smile." Other common descriptions I have heard include "toothy" and "horsey." An example of what most orthodontists would consider a protrusive smile is shown in Figures 10.2a and 10.2b. Notice also that the patient must strain to close her lips together. This lip strain is another indication that the smile is excessively protrusive.

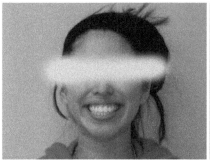 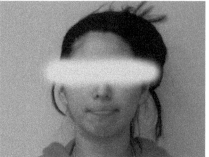

Figures 10.2a and 10.2b

When orthodontists evaluate patients with severe crowding, they must always decide about whether or not to take teeth out. Patients and their parents should always be a part of this discussion. Many times, I have had patients and parents seek a second opinion with me because their orthodontist placed braces on them, and later in treatment informed them that they should have had teeth taken out. Patients and parents are understandably surprised and dismayed when this discussion occurs halfway through their orthodontic treatment. Parents and patients should always be told up front whether the orthodontist believes adult teeth should be removed as part of the overall treatment plan. Even if the orthodontist feels the patient is a "borderline" case for extraction, the orthodontist should inform the patient and parent up front prior to treatment and discuss the progress at each adjustment appointment until a definitive decision is reached.

OTHER REASONS WHY ADULT TOOTH REMOVAL MAY BE NECESSARY

In addition to severe crowding reasons, there are other instances in which an orthodontist may recommend the removal of adult teeth as part of treatment.

MISMATCHED JAWS

If a patient has mismatched jaws, the ideal treatment is usually to reposition the jaws surgically. Most people, given a choice, would rather avoid jaw surgery, however. Fortunately, in most patients, excellent results can be achieved with the removal of adult teeth to help resolve the mismatch without surgery. Patients with a large upper jaw in relation to a smaller lower jaw oftentimes have an excessive overbite. Adult teeth in the upper jaw can be removed to help fix an overbite. Patients with a larger lower jaw in relation to a smaller upper jaw oftentimes have an underbite. Adult teeth in the lower jaw can be removed to help fix an underbite. The decision to remove adult teeth as an alternative to surgically repositioning the jaws should be discussed by patients, parents, and the orthodontist prior to proceeding with treatment.

COSMETIC REASONS

Another reason why an orthodontist may recommend or agree with the removal of adult teeth is largely cosmetic. Sometimes patients have protrusive smiles with minimal to no crowding. Quite often, these patients have done their homework and come to their first appointment with me to tell me they want teeth taken out to make their smile better and their lip profile flatter. This scenario (the occurrence of and request for removal of adult teeth) is more common in my patients of Asian, Hispanic, and African American ethnicity. An example of a patient with minimal crowding and a protrusive smile that was improved to her liking is shown in the photo collage below. See Figures 10.3 and 10.4.

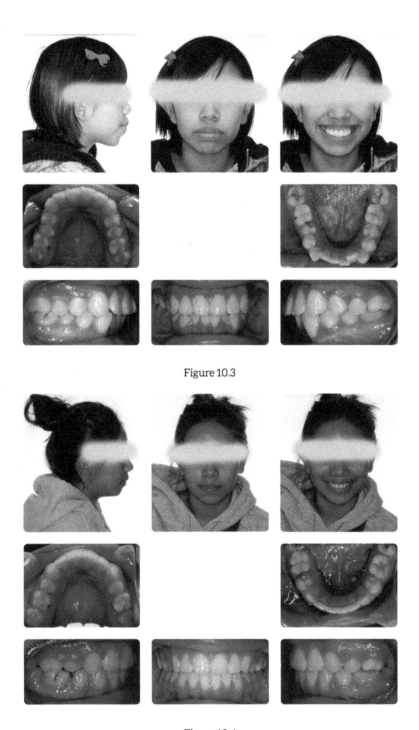

Figure 10.3

Figure 10.4

TOOTH REMOVAL CAN BE AVOIDED (IN MOST CASES)

Now it is time to get back to the fact that, in most cases, tooth removal can be avoided. So, if you think you may need adult teeth taken out, do not despair. The first step is to schedule an exam with an orthodontist. The need to take out teeth for orthodontic treatment nowadays is exceedingly low compared to days past.

Personally, I treat hundreds of patients every year and I come across fewer than five patients each year who I feel should have adult teeth taken out as part of their treatment.

Most patients who are told they need to have adult teeth removed often seek multiple opinions. And they should. The removal of teeth adds to the expense of orthodontic treatment, and there is a period of healing afterward that must be managed with pain medication. Also, once they are removed, adult teeth do not grow back. You want to make sure you are doing the right thing. If you get multiple, reputable opinions and they are all telling you that you should have adult teeth removed, then you can at least put your mind at ease about the best path forward. If some orthodontists are telling you that you should have teeth removed and others are not, then you will have to decide which path to take. I will tell you what I always tell patients who come to me for first, second, or even third opinions—when you are in this situation, ask whichever orthodontist you choose to start treatment without taking out the adult teeth, provided it will not jeopardize the health of the teeth. Then, have the orthodontist tell you when the teeth are fully aligned. If you like the way your smile looks, then leave the teeth in. If you don't like your smile and feel it is "toothy," then have the adult teeth taken out. It may lengthen your overall time in braces by a couple of months, but you'll be more confident that you made the right decision and you will get the smile you've always wanted.

chapter eleven

THE IMPORTANCE OF RETAINING YOUR RETAINER

So, the braces are off, and you are free from the need to use any appliances on your teeth ever again. Not so fast.

A retainer is necessary to keep your teeth from shifting and becoming crooked again. Orthodontists may have varying opinions on how often to wear the retainers, but all agree that retainers must be worn after braces or Invisalign. This is a fact backed up by a lot of research.[27]

Another little-known fact is that people who are born with naturally straight teeth and never had to wear braces as teenagers should also wear retainers at least part-time to hold their current teeth positions. Teeth shift slowly over time and throughout our

---

27   M. Blake and K. Bibby, "Retention and Stability: A Review of the Literature," *Am J of Orthod and Dentofacial Orthop* 114, no. 3 (1998): 299-306, https://doi.org/10.1016/S0889-5406(98)70212-4

lives.[28] Teeth tend to get more crowded as we age, especially the lower front teeth. However, in people who grind and clench their teeth, the teeth tend to space apart. Other conditions, like periodontal disease and teeth extraction, can accelerate the shifting process. This shifting of the teeth is a natural part of the aging process, just like getting gray hairs or wrinkles, and the only way to prevent it is by wearing retainers part-time.

Later in this chapter, we will discuss the perils of not wearing your retainers after finishing treatment with braces or Invisalign, and how long you should wear your retainers, but first, let's talk about the types of retainers available today.

TYPES OF RETAINERS

There are basically three kinds of retainers, including fixed retainers, Hawley retainers, and vacuum-formed retainers.

FIXED RETAINERS

Fixed retainers are permanent and cannot be removed for eating and brushing the teeth. Other names for fixed retainers include bonded retainers and permanent retainers. A fixed retainer is simply a metal wire that is glued to the back of the teeth. It can be glued to the upper and/or lower front teeth. However, fixed retainers are more often used on the lower teeth than the upper teeth, because upper fixed retainers are more susceptible to breaking.

Fixed retainers are only visible by the patient and only when looking in a mirror. Some parents prefer fixed retainers because they are concerned that their children would not wear the removable type.

---

28   Ibid.; Robert M. Little, "Stability and Relapse of Dental Arch Alignment," *British Journal of Orthodontics* 22, no. 3 (1995): 235-241, https://doi.org/10.1179/bjo.17.3

With fixed retainers, their children do not have the option of taking out their retainers and losing them.

A primary disadvantage of fixed retainers is patients have difficulty keeping their teeth clean. Brushing and flossing around a fixed retainer takes some practice and is not as simple as removing a retainer to brush and floss the teeth. Another disadvantage to fixed retainers, especially fixed retainers for the upper teeth, is that they are known to break from time to time. Most orthodontists will charge $50 to $300 to repair or replace broken fixed retainers. For this reason, I steer patients away from upper fixed retainers because of the frequent need for repair and/or replacement. Lower fixed retainers can last decades and are usually more cost effective. A picture of fixed retainer placed on the lower teeth is shown below (Figure 11.1).

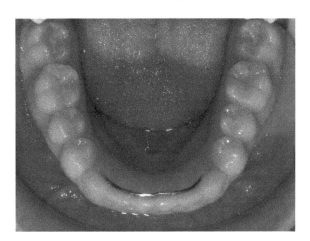

Figure 11.1

HAWLEY RETAINER

The second type of retainer, a Hawley retainer, is a more traditional type of retainer that you may have seen children wearing. These retainers have a clear or gum-colored plastic that covers the palette, and a metal wire that runs around the front of the teeth. Hawley retainers are very durable and can last a lifetime if they are well cared for and not stepped on, driven over by a car, or chewed up by a dog. Hawley retainers have a longer shelf-life if they are stored in their case and taken in and out properly. A child is prone to dislike the metal wire that runs along the front of the teeth. Teenagers have told me the only thing cooler than wearing this type of retainer is wearing braces (insert sarcasm). Replacements or repairs to Hawley retainers typically run $50 to $300. Patients tend to misplace the removable Hawley retainers. An example of a Hawley retainer is shown in the next two photographs (Figure 11.2a and 11.2b).

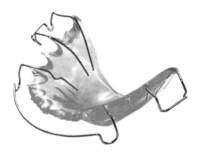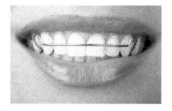

Figures 11.2a and 11.2b

VACUUM-FORMED RETAINER

The third type of retainer available is called a vacuum-formed retainer. Other terms for this type of retainer are Essix retainer and invisible retainer. These retainers have become more popular in recent years because they are easy to make and patients generally approve of the way they look. When a vacuum-formed retainer is being worn, it looks very similar to Invisalign; that is, it is invisible. You can't see it unless you're very, very close to a person and looking right at their teeth. These retainers are like Hawley retainers in that you can take them out to eat and to brush and floss. One advantage of the vacuum-formed retainer is that if you do lose or break it, they are a little less expensive to replace compared to a fixed or Hawley retainer. Replacement costs for vacuum-formed retainers typically run $75 to $200. However, if these retainers are damaged, they usually cannot be repaired. The main disadvantage to vacuum-formed retainers is that they are more delicate than Hawley retainers. They tend to crack and break if not taken in and out carefully. If you grind and clench your teeth at night like many people do, they tend to get holes in them and break down even quicker. On average, vacuum-formed retainers only last six months to two years. Since they have become more popular in recent years, some orthodontists now offer unlimited replacements for a yearly fee that is more cost effective than paying for them every time they crack, break, or wear out. A vacuum-formed retainer is shown in the following two photographs (Figure 11.3a and 11.3b).

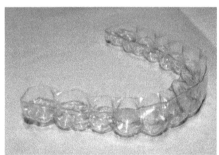 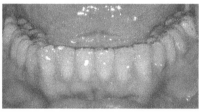

Figure 11.3a and 11.3b

WHAT HAPPENS IF YOU DON'T WEAR YOUR RETAINER

Now that we know all the facts, and the advantages and disadvantages about the types of retainers available, it's time to answer the question, "What happens if I don't wear my retainer? (or my child doesn't?)" The truth is, nothing positive can result. Ok, that is a bit flippant, but it is the truth.

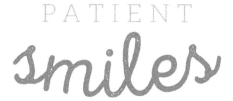PATIENT *smiles*

I had braces in fifth grade to straighten my front teeth, and then a full set of braces and headgear in high school. When I went to college, I lost my retainer and didn't go get a replacement. So, as an adult my overbite returned, and my bottom and top teeth were starting to turn and move out of place. In addition, my bite was off; this was causing me to grind my teeth at night, which resulted in a lot of pain.

So, I went in for an assessment with Dr. Verbic and had a great experience. They estimated about a year in braces and it took about ten months. I was diligent about wearing the rubber bands, which helped, I think. Then I spent about ten or eleven months wearing the clear retainer full time. And now I'm just wearing the night time retainer and will continue to wear it this time, so my teeth don't move back!

I had a wonderful experience with Dr. Verbic and his staff. I loved going in for my checkups. Everyone was so nice and they made a point to get to know me. It was like going in to see friends each time. I'll be honest, while I don't miss the braces, I do miss going in to see the Verbic team! **—LAUREN H.**

For patients who have recently had orthodontic treatment, their teeth are not accustomed to their new positions in their jawbone. My analogy: it can be compared to teeth floating in a soupy concrete that has not been set. They are very prone to unwanted shifting during this time. Orthodontic research has shown that it takes approximately seven to eight months after braces have been removed for the teeth to set in their new positions.[29] If patients don't wear their retainers during this time, then it is very likely that the teeth will shift, sometimes dramatically, and patients often require additional time back in braces or Invisalign. This is not only an unnecessary financial burden, but it is also a social and time burden. I understand the desire for minimal effort and intrusion in daily routines, but unfortunately, we don't have a magic wand that says, "Teeth, stay here." We do have retainers and they DO work in keeping teeth in position. We hate seeing former patients come back in several years after their initial treatment needing additional treatment. Is it good to see them on a personal level? Absolutely. Can we fix their teeth again? Absolutely. Does our practice earn more money? Yes. Do we take pleasure in earning more money in these cases? Absolutely not. Please, please wear your retainer.

HOW LONG IS IT NECESSARY TO WEAR YOUR RETAINER?

We all understand the importance of wearing a retainer after initially finishing treatment with braces or Invisalign. But, a question that I'm asked practically every day at work is, "How *long* do I have to wear my retainer?" The short answer to that is, "For the rest of your life, but only if you want to keep your teeth straight." As we discussed above, research has shown that it takes about eight months after braces have been removed for the teeth to set in their new positions.[30]

The vacuum-formed retainers can be worn by most people part-time (while sleeping) right away because they are flexible and

---

29 K. Reitan, "Clinical and Histologic Observations on Tooth Movement During and After Orthodontic Treatment," *Am J Orthod* 53, no. 10 (1967) 721–45, https://doi. org/10.1016/0002-9416(67)90118-2; J. G. Edwards, "A Study of the Periodontium During Orthodontic Rotation of Teeth," *Am J of Ortho* 54, no. 6 (1968): 441–61, https://doi.org/10.1016/0002-9416(68)90199-1

30 Ibid.

can realign teeth that have moved a minor amount during the day. Some people have teeth that relapse more right away and cannot just wear their vacuum-formed retainers at night. Orthodontists cannot distinguish between those that can and those that cannot get away with part-time wear right after treatment. Most orthodontists ask their patients to wear them full-time immediately after treatment.

So, it is *VERY* important for patients to wear their retainers full time (during the day and night) for those first several months. After this time, and especially after the first year, teeth are much more stable, but they can still move. Therefore, orthodontists recommend patients still wear retainers part-time, usually every night (while they are sleeping) for life, to keep their teeth straight.

I often see a disappointed look on my patients' faces when I advise them this way, but it is important to look at this from a different perspective. What other beauty-enhancing procedure can you have performed just one time and it lasts for the rest of your life? Botox injections will reduce wrinkles, but only for a few months. Even, if you have plastic surgery, like a facelift, there is no retainer to keep the results over time. You can pretty much count on having to do that same surgery ten or fifteen years down the road as you continue to age. After investing in braces or Invisalign treatment, all you must do is wear your retainers at night, if they are removable, or spend a little more time brushing and flossing around fixed retainers. This is all you need to do to preserve your perfect smile for the rest of your life and you'll never have to have braces or Invisalign again!

chapter twelve

DON'T WORRY SO MUCH ABOUT WISDOM TEETH

Wisdom teeth, technically called the third set of molars, usually erupt in the mouth starting in the teen years, but they are potentially still developing in young adults in their twenties or even thirties. Due to the timing of the eruption of these teeth, I see a lot of patients who are concerned about them. I hear the following questions a lot:

- "Are my wisdom teeth impacted or not impacted, and what does that actually mean?"

- "Will I need to get my wisdom teeth removed?"

- "If I keep them, will they cause my teeth to shift after my braces are off?"

These are all good questions. The first question about the difference between non-impacted and impacted wisdom teeth is easy to answer. Non-impacted wisdom teeth are teeth that have fully erupted within the mouth. They have the appearance of a normal molar. Impacted wisdom teeth are teeth that have not erupted out the jaw bone at all and remain embedded. There is a third category, in which they are partially impacted. Partially impacted wisdom teeth are teeth that have started to erupt out of the jaw bone and are partially in the mouth; usually showing through the gum tissue, but not fully erupted.

Many patients ask if they should have their wisdom teeth removed. The answer depends on whether they are impacted. Even then, there is controversy.

The next couple of sections will address this question.

Patients are relieved to learn that the eruption of their wisdom teeth will not cause teeth to shift and interfere with orthodontic work.

NON-IMPACTED WISDOM TEETH

In most situations, but with a lot of caveats, people with non-impacted wisdom teeth can keep their teeth. I am one of those people.

> When I was growing up I remember my older brother and his friends having their wisdom teeth taken out. It seemed like a rite of passage for everyone in his or her late teens to early twenties, and it was something that I was not looking forward to.
>
> Fortunately, my wisdom teeth were not impacted, and my childhood dentist did not recommend their removal. However, as I got into my mid-to-late twenties, my dentist became more concerned with the health of my wisdom teeth and the teeth next to them, the second molars. It seems that I was not doing a good enough job brushing and flossing them. Like most people, I was not very good at getting a toothbrush and floss back that far in my mouth. My dentist told me if I did not improve at keeping my wisdom teeth clean, that I would have to have them taken out. Through diligent home care and

> *keeping up with my dental cleanings every six months, I have been able to keep my wisdom teeth, and keep them healthy.*
>
> **—DR. VERBIC**

Because I work frequently with teenagers, I relay my story to those with wisdom teeth that are coming in correctly. I do not recommend wisdom teeth be removed, as long as the patients are able and willing to practice high-quality dental hygiene by brushing and flossing them twice per day. However, I emphasize that this dental hygiene is essential, but difficult, and that they must be committed to taking care of these teeth. Many don't understand the critical importance of taking care of the wisdom teeth, and they don't understand how difficult it can be to keep them clean. If a person does a poor job in keeping the wisdom teeth clean, big problems can result.

Non-impacted wisdom teeth are prone to cavities. This is especially true for partially impacted wisdom teeth. Because these teeth are partially within the gums, food can get caught easily and it is difficult to floss in these cases.

Wisdom teeth are difficult to take care of because they are far back in the mouth. It can be quite difficult to reach the wisdom teeth, and people are usually not good about getting the toothbrush and floss back there. I understand; I am a dentist and it is difficult for me to get the floss back there. In addition, the older you get, the less well your hands work and the more difficult it is to maneuver the toothbrush and floss back there. Many people think that they are adequately cleaning their wisdom teeth, when in reality, they are not.

The timing of wisdom teeth eruption, combined with poor dental hygiene, often coincides with teenagers going off to college or dropping off their parents' dental insurance. A significant lapse in regular visits occurs.

My twin brother's story is a cautionary tale of what happens when you don't take good care of your non-impacted wisdom teeth.

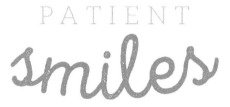

PATIENT *smiles*

When my twin brother, Marty, was in his orthodontic residency program after having earned his dental degree and obtaining his dental license, he was moonlighting as a dentist on the weekends to pay down student debt from dental school. As soon as he started working, friends and family members asked him to help them out; partly because they trusted him, but also because he could fix their dental problems for free. Well, I was one of those family members who asked for help. Like Marty, I kept my wisdom teeth because they were not impacted, but I had a big problem with one of my wisdom teeth. I had a filling on my upper-left wisdom tooth that had gone bad. I could feel a hole in my tooth with my tongue! I knew it was bad and begged Marty to help me out. He told me that if I felt a hole, it was probably going to be a pretty bad case.

He leaned me back in the dental chair and looked inside my mouth. He said, "Oh yeah, I see a big crater in the tooth; a huge cavity." He told me that he honestly didn't think he would be able to fix it. He told me that the tooth should probably be taken out. Well, I started begging him to fix the tooth and not take it out, and my amazing brother gave in to my pleading and got to work trying to save my tooth.

He tried his best, but the work was beyond his capability at the time. Thankfully, the senior dentist at his practice was nice and volunteered to jump in and finish the procedure to fix and save my tooth. That day, I learned a very difficult and important lesson about getting the toothbrush and floss back there to clean my wisdom teeth. I know that this is the only way I will continue to be able to keep that tooth and my other wisdom teeth as I get older. **—VICTOR VERBIC**

Not everyone is as fortunate as my brother. Many people have healthy wisdom teeth, but since cavities are an infection, the problems can spread in their mouth to other teeth. It is the same story with periodontal disease and bone loss. If it affects the wisdom teeth, then it can also affect the second molars next to them. It is kind of like a snowball effect, all really caused by these wisdom teeth.

Therefore, I am biased. I advise patients who have not demonstrated healthy maintenance habits to have their wisdom teeth removed to prevent causing problems later in life. Younger people can recover from surgery better and it is less intrusive in their lives. If wisdom teeth are removed, there is no more worry about the possibility of a tooth becoming infected while on a vacation, which could turn into a major problem.

So, in the end, for non-impacted wisdom teeth, keeping them is fine "as long as you are 100 percent committed to taking very good care of them. It is a big commitment and shouldn't be taken lightly.

For those with impacted wisdom teeth, however, the situation isn't as clear cut."

IMPACTED WISDOM TEETH

There is a fair amount of controversy in the dental field today about whether all impacted wisdom teeth should be removed. Some experts believe that all impacted wisdom teeth should be removed, whereas other experts believe only impacted wisdom teeth that are causing pain or infection should be removed.[31] Basically, there is a non-removal camp and a removal camp.

---

31   Dirk Mettes et al. "Interventions for treating asymptomatic impacted wisdom teeth in adolescents and adults," *Cochrane Database of Systematic Reviews*, no. 2 (2005), https://doi.org/10.1002/14651858.CD003879.pub2

As stated earlier, both sides agree that wisdom teeth *do not* contribute to crowding or movement of other teeth that have been straightened by braces. As you can imagine, parents are usually relieved when I inform them that the eruption of their child's wisdom teeth *will not* ruin their child's orthodontic result.

NON-REMOVAL CAMP

The experts that believe impacted teeth should not be removed unless they are causing problems; reason that the risks of their removal outweigh the risks of leaving them in place. Since patients are usually anesthetized prior to wisdom tooth removal, there is always the small chance that they may not wake up from the surgery. Across all surgeries performed across the United States, however, the mortality rate for dental surgery is minimal, at three deaths for every 1 million anesthetic administrations.[32] With every surgery, there is also the risk of infection. Antibiotics are usually prescribed as a precaution after all wisdom tooth removal surgeries, however, to minimize the chance for infection. There is also the risk of damage to surrounding structures, such as other teeth, nerves, and bones, when wisdom teeth are removed. The risk of damage to surrounding structures, fortunately, is small.

Both your orthodontist and the oral surgeon removing your or your child's wisdom teeth should take the time to discuss the benefits and possible complications associated with the procedure.

REMOVAL CAMP

The experts who believe that all impacted wisdom teeth should be removed reason that, if left in place, wisdom teeth will eventually

---

32   G. Li et al., "Epidemiology of Anesthesia-Related Mortality in the United States, 1999–2005," *Anesthesiology* 4, no. 110 (2009): 759–65, https://doi.org/10.1097/ALN.0b013e31819b5bdc

cause problems somewhere down the road. Impacted wisdom teeth often cause pain and swelling when they try to erupt into the mouth. It is advised to remove them before the pain and swelling occur. Also, when wisdom teeth must be removed later in life—when people are in their thirties, forties, or fifties, for instance—the healing process can take longer and be more difficult in general. In short, what is the message? "Spontaneous cystic changes in impacted wisdom teeth are uncommon, but can cause severe jaw infection and destruction of bone." And, finally, when wisdom teeth erupt, but are poorly positioned, they can be virtually impossible to brush and floss adequately. This can lead to cavities and periodontal disease on both the wisdom teeth and the second molars, next to them.

LAST WORD ON THE MATTER

Current research is not conclusive on whether impacted wisdom teeth should be removed to prevent possible future problems or not.[33] Based on my own professional experience and that of other dental professionals, I *do* recommend the removal of most impacted wisdom teeth in my patients because of the problems I have seen them cause later in life. But, if you do not wish to have your or your child's wisdom teeth removed, that is ok too. If this is the route you choose, you should ask your family dentist about the status of the wisdom teeth at each of your six-month examination and cleaning appointments.

So, now that you know you don't have to worry too much about wisdom teeth, let's move on to another topic that is a frequent cause of unnecessary worry: the costs for orthodontic treatment. You will

---

33 Theodorus Mettes et al., "Surgical Removal Versus Retention for the Management of Asymptomatic Impacted Wisdom Teeth," *Cochrane Database of Symptomatic Reviews* 6 (June 2012), https://doi.org/10.1002/14651858.CD003879.pub3

soon see that you don't need to worry too much about this topic, either. Asking good questions, doing your research and careful planning are the keys to stress-free financial management of orthodontic treatment.

chapter thirteen

PAYING FOR ORTHODONTIC TREATMENT: IT DOESN'T HAVE TO BREAK THE BANK

There is no question that quality orthodontic treatment is expensive. It is a significant financial investment in yourself or your child. However, it is also an investment in your or your child's physical, emotional, and psychological health. In fact, you can't afford NOT to do this. The benefits to your or your child's life far outweigh the financial cost. Today, the payment options available are different from what they used to be and, though expensive, quality orthodontic treatment can be quite affordable. In fact, it is relatively easy to put together a well-thought-out financial plan through payment options, orthodontic insurance, and HSAs or FSAs. This chapter will give you the information you need to start putting your financial plan together.

ORTHODONTIC TREATMENT IS MORE AFFORDABLE THAN YOU THINK

Paying for orthodontic treatment is easier today than at any point in the past. The inflation-adjusted average cost of braces has fallen since the 1960s, mostly due to technological advances in the field. The average cost of braces today is around $6,000, but the cost can range from as little as $250 for an aligner to move a tooth slightly, to more than $40,000 if jaw surgery is needed.[34] Therefore, it is advisable to have an exam or consultation first to find out what is needed. The good news is that most orthodontists offer free exams and consultations so that you can find out exactly how much braces will cost for you or your children. Most orthodontists recognize how important a straight smile is in our society and they will do everything possible to help parents and children to get started. The best orthodontic practices have expert staff who know the ins and outs of financing, orthodontic insurance, and HSAs and FSAs. This staff will work with each patient in helping them put together the financial plan that works best for them.

FINANCING FACTS

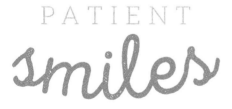

PATIENT
smiles

I have worked in orthodontics for twenty-five years and it is amazing how much paying for orthodontic treatment has changed over the years; especially big changes have occurred within the last two to three years. It is not only financing that has changed, it is also the communication between our office and our patients that has changed.

---

34 "How Much Do Braces Cost?" BracesInfo, www.bracesinfo.com/how-much-do-braces-cost.html?_ga=2.195537962.782868287.1511801806-951462198. 1511801806

In the past, people had to put down a 25 to 30 percent down-payment and had to finish paying it off during treatment time—no exceptions. Today, we open up a line of communication with each new patient. Of course, we love to get a 20 to 30 percent down-payment, but we do not hold people to this. We talk with each patient about how to make payments fit their budget. We work with our patients to make a payment schedule to work for them financially. Today, the average financing is about thirty to forty-eight months, which often goes beyond treatment time. Of course, we do a background check, but with the advent of auto drafting of payments, the fear that patients won't pay is lessened.

It can be very difficult for patients to admit in person they can't afford orthodontic treatment. If, during our first meeting, I sense this is the case for patients, I always get them back on the phone for follow up with questions. On the phone, they are more comfortable and better able to tell me what they can afford financially. We work it out, devise a payment plan, and then they schedule treatment. This communication helps to break down barriers, and helps people feel comfortable, which then leads them to schedule treatment.

Our office policies have led to increased communication with our very happy patients who are not as stressed about paying for orthodontic treatment. Also, due to our policies, fewer people seek a second opinion due to cost or financing after talking to us. **—LORI H., TREATMENT COORDINATOR AT VERBIC ORTHODONTICS**

Years ago, orthodontic treatment was reserved for those who were relatively wealthy, because a typical financing plan for paying for orthodontic treatment was to pay a 25 percent down-payment before starting treatment, and then the entire cost had to be paid within the two years. But nobody walks around with $2,000 in their pocket anymore. Most orthodontic practices have evolved in their financing plans to adapt to changes in financial culture, but also to make orthodontic treatment more affordable for more people. Financing has become the key for everything. We just had a patient last week who couldn't put anything down and wanted to pay $100 a month for five years and our finance department said, "Okay, this plan will work." Today's common financing options are flexible and often tailored toward a patient's terms and their ability to pay.

Orthodontists understand that patients come to us because they really want to fix their or their child's teeth. It is not like they are not going to pay us. The orthodontic practices that are smart understand this, and their practices thrive and can help more patients afford quality orthodontic treatment. The orthodontic practices that are worried patients are going to rip them off if the financing plan is too generous don't understand how a business works.

For instance, orthodontic practices will offer zero-interest financing for at least twenty-four months and some will even offer no down-payment to make treatment more affordable. After the insurance benefit (see the next section), a typical payment plan includes payments of less than $200 per month. And unlike your cable bill or family cell phone bill, those payments will end after twenty-four months and you'll get to enjoy the confidence of a straight smile for the rest of your life.

ORTHODONTIC INSURANCE

Orthodontic insurance assists in making treatment financially viable. Orthodontic insurance is a benefit that parents and patients may have, but do not understand. Or, some people might not know orthodontic insurance is even available, think it will be too expensive and not worth it, or assume it will be included in dental insurance plans. I understand. I don't even fully understand my own medical insurance when I go to see my doctor. Fortunately, most orthodontic offices will help you understand what it is and how it works. If you have orthodontic insurance, they will help you get your full benefit. In fact, it is in the orthodontic office's best financial interest and their relationship with you to help you maximize your insurance benefit.

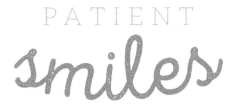

One of the best examples of how our office staff can help to make orthodontic insurance work for our patients is exemplified by a family that had two children who both required two phases of treatment. Both parents worked and both had orthodontic insurance, but they were nervous about how to best utilize their existing insurance. We sat with this family to look at the policies and figure out with them that the best way to utilize the insurance benefit would be to use one parent's insurance benefit for phase 1 treatment and to use the other parent's insurance benefit for phase 2 treatment. The family also had Flexible Savings Accounts. Using the money from these accounts, combined with their insurance benefits, resulted in this family barely having to pay much out of pocket. It took some effort to figure it all out, but they were so thankful and happy with our office that they told all their friends, family, and colleagues about Verbic Orthodontics. This story is a great example of why I love what I do. **—LORI H., TREATMENT COORDINATOR AT VERBIC ORTHODONTICS**

In my experience, people are very familiar with their dental insurance, but not as much with their orthodontic insurance. With dental insurance, every year patients first must meet their deductible. Then, for the remainder of that calendar year, they're covered at about 80 to 90 percent of the cost of treatment if they go to a doctor in their network. Patients are then responsible for paying the remaining 10 to 20 percent themselves out of their own pocket. If they go to an out-of-network doctor, their benefit may only be 50 percent, on average.

Orthodontic insurance is a lot different than dental insurance and it is always listed as a separate benefit. The biggest differences are discussed below.

NOT ALL DENTAL INSURANCE PLANS INCLUDE ORTHODONTICS

This is a very important point that every parent and patient should be aware of and should think about at least a year before considering beginning orthodontic treatment. It is important to plan when you think orthodontic treatment is a possibility for yourself or your child. Our office has had patients come in and say to us, "Ok, we are ready to start treatment and we have insurance." Our office personnel must break the bad news that their dental plan does not include orthodontic coverage. Many say, "I didn't realize that the cheaper dental plan I signed up for at the office doesn't include orthodontics." These families then must wait an entire year before they can opt into the more-expensive plan that includes orthodontic insurance. This delay can be quite detrimental to patients. For example, the parents may have timed it so that their child would complete orthodontic treatment before starting high school. Or, the delay in starting treatment might result in the child reaching a possible age limit (see below) to use the insurance payment; once their child reaches this age limit, the insurance company will not pay. Therefore, it is vital to plan at least a year ahead and choose the best policy with the best orthodontic coverage possible.

LIFETIME MAXIMUM BENEFIT

One of the primary differences between dental and orthodontic insurance is that there is a lifetime maximum amount that the insurance will pay for orthodontic treatment. This amount usually ranges from $1,000 benefit on the low-end to potentially as high as

$2,500 per lifetime, per family member. This can be confusing to parents and patients; insurance companies will only pay out up to the lifetime maximum amount for orthodontic treatment even if two phases of treatment are needed and it's in the patient's best interests. If the insurance company has already paid out the entire lifetime maximum amount for the first phase of treatment (as is usually the case), they will not pay again several years later when the patient is ready for the second phase of treatment. Parents and patients are free to change insurances and get another lifetime maximum benefit for the second phase of treatment, but since most people get insurance through their workplace it is usually not possible or practical to change to a different insurance company. Occasionally, parents will purchase two separate policies, however insurance companies will only allow one policy to pay at a time. By the time treatment is finished, it is rare that both policies lifetime maximum amounts can be fully utilized. The exception is with treatment that occurs in two phases. If this is the case, both policies can usually be fully utilized.

Another source of confusion is how the insurance company pays out the lifetime maximum amount. Parents and patients sometimes think that the insurance company will pay the entire amount when treatment begins. But this is never the case. This can be a major disappointment to parents and patients who attempted to use the insurance to pay for the down-payment that may be required at some orthodontic offices. Unfortunately, the lifetime maximum amount is paid slowly over the course of treatment. The orthodontic office must submit an orthodontic claim once a month to the insurance company letting them know that the orthodontic treatment is still underway and being provided. The insurance company will then send payment to the office either once a month or once a quarter until the lifetime maximum amount is reached.

IN-NETWORK PROVIDERS VERSUS OUT-OF-NETWORK PROVIDERS

The other major difference between dental insurances and orthodontic insurances is that orthodontic insurances will usually pay the same lifetime maximum amount whether you go to an in-network provider or out-of-network provider. Remember that for dental insurances, the amount that the insurance will cover for an out-of-network provider is substantially less than they will cover for an in-network provider. With some orthodontic insurance policies, the benefit may be reduced from $500-$1000, but this is rare. The vast majority of policies will pay the same amount. In many instances, however, in-network orthodontic offices will charge substantially less for treatment than will out-of-network orthodontic offices. This is because the in-network offices have entered into a contract with the insurance company and have agreed not to charge patients more than a certain amount for treatment, in exchange for being included in that insurance company's list of orthodontic offices that they provide to their patients. The out-of-network providers are not included in this list.

As you can imagine, this is an effective means of advertising to obtain more patients for the in-network orthodontic practices. The drawback for the in-network offices is that they must reduce their fees substantially, sometimes by up to 40 percent. This seems like a great deal for patients, but the in-network offices must make up for the shortfall in fees somehow, or they will go bankrupt and out of business. They will usually make up for the shortfall by treating a higher volume of patients. This may make it more difficult for patients to get appointments at the times and days that they would like. It may make treatment more hurried and inaccurate as well, as the office must process more patients through the office on any given day. Other ways to make up for the shortfall in fees include charging extra for clear treatment options like ceramic braces or Invisalign, charging for missed or late appointments, charging for treatment that takes longer than a given period (usually twenty-four months), charging inflated prices for lost or broken retainers, and charging extra for appliances like expanders that are not necessary.

The level of customer service usually suffers as well, because the office has a hard time paying for enough staff to answer telephone calls and helping patients to understand their treatment, insurance, and payments. You've likely experienced this already if you've gone to a medical doctor in the last fifteen years. It is not uncommon to wait thirty minutes to an hour for a scheduled appointment and the support staff can be less than helpful. Emergency room waits can take up to twenty-four hours. At the end of the day, it is possible to pay more in extra fees, lost time, and having to redo orthodontic treatment again due to poor treatment the first time than it would have cost to go to reputable office that may be out of network. Kurt Vonnegut's (*Cat's Cradle*) old saying, "In the world, you get what you pay for," holds true. Unfortunately, patients will sometimes gravitate toward the lowest-cost orthodontic office, not realizing that it will end up costing them more in the long run. It can be much wiser to look for the best value and not necessarily the lowest price, as with most things in life.

COVERAGE FOR ADULT PATIENTS

We advise that you verify your insurance policy prior to beginning treatment. Some insurance policies do not cover adult orthodontic treatment, so if you plan to have treatment and you are an adult you should check your policy or have the orthodontic office verify your coverage before beginning treatment. Orthodontic insurance policies often restrict the patient's age limit for treatment to nineteen years.

It also means that if a patient is currently in treatment, the insurance company will stop paying once the patient turns nineteen years of age. This can be a real disappointment to parents and patients, so it is better to know this upfront before orthodontic treatment begins. Some insurance companies are recognizing that children live with their parents longer and are still dependents, so they have raised the age limit to as high as twenty-six in some instances, but the vast majority of insurance companies still use nineteen as the age limit. Some insurance policies may cover your spouse as well, so if your spouse is interested in treatment you should check your policy or have the orthodontic office verify if there is coverage.

WAITING PERIODS

Finally, you will also want to be aware of any waiting periods on your insurance policy. The waiting period is the time between when you buy the policy and when the orthodontic treatment begins. Some policies take effect immediately and have no waiting period, while others have waiting periods of thirty, sixty, or ninety days. If you begin treatment before the waiting period has ended, you may end up receiving a reduced benefit or, in extreme circumstances, no benefit at all. Also, if the insurance policy ends for any reason (like the loss of a job), then you will be responsible for paying any amount that the insurance company did not pay the orthodontic office.

HSAs AND FSAs AND HOW THEY SAVE YOU MONEY

Health Savings Accounts (HSAs) and Flexible Spending Accounts (FSAs) are accounts that allow parents and patients to set aside money tax-fee to use on qualified medical expenses. Parents can use their HSAs or FSAs for orthodontic treatment for themselves or for their children. The biggest difference between HSAs and FSAs is that if you don't spend the money that you put into an FSA in each calendar year, you lose it. Some FSAs now allow you to carry over $500 per year, but any amount more than $500 will still be forfeited if you don't use it. The money that you put into an HSA, on the other hand, is yours forever. The money that you put into an HSA can also be invested in a manner like an IRA and, just like an IRA, the money continues to grow tax free. Once you reach age sixty-five, or if you become disabled, you may withdraw money from your HSA even if it is not for qualified medical expenses and pay only ordinary income tax. If you withdraw money from your HSA prior to age sixty-five for any reason other than qualified medical expenses, you will have to pay ordinary income tax plus a 20 percent penalty. For 2017, the most that you can put in to an HSA is $3,400 for yourself or $6,750 for your family. For FSAs, as of 2017, the most that you may put in per year is $2,600.[35]

Your orthodontic practice will provide you with receipts or any other documentation that may be required by your HSA or FSA as proof that the money in the accounts is being used for a qualified medical expense. The amount that you can save on orthodontic treatment depends on your income tax rate. If, for example, your overall income tax rate is 20 percent, then you will essentially be saving 20 percent on your orthodontic treatment if you pay for all your treatment with funds from your HSA and/or FSA. Depending on the orthodontic practice and how long your treatment takes, you may also be able to arrange to use two consecutive years of HSA and FSA benefits. When you combine these savings with any insurance benefits, orthodontic treatment becomes even more affordable.

---

35   "Publication 969 (2016), Health Savings Accounts and Other Tax-Favored Health Plans," IRS, https://www.irs.gov/publications/p969

We covered a lot of important, and somewhat technical, information about the finances of orthodontic treatment. As mentioned earlier, finding a great practice that has a highly-qualified billing department really can make the difference as you wade through the finances of paying for orthodontic treatment. Their expert advice combined with your own careful planning really will take the stress out of the whole process. Don't worry.

chapter fourteen

WHEN YOU REALLY CAN'T AFFORD TREATMENT FOR YOUR CHILD

> *One of my strongest passions as an orthodontist is to make sure that children whose parents can't afford the cost of orthodontic treatment have access to treatment. Every child should have the right to a beautiful smile. Really, it all comes down to one thing: Creating a confidant smile in as many patients as possible.*
>
> **—DR. VERBIC**

As discussed in the last chapter, thankfully, orthodontic treatment payment terms have become achievable and more flexible today. However, this is obviously not financially possible for many families. When a family is faced with choosing between safe housing or nutritious food and orthodontic treatment for their child, braces are not going to win. However—and this is where I will start to get emotional about my passion for orthodontics—this doesn't necessarily have to be the case. This chapter is important, not only for readers who are in this financial situation, but for all families out there. My mission is to raise awareness of this issue; I want others to share information on this topic (and perhaps donate to worthy causes). Together, we can make a difference in helping families who really can't afford orthodontic treatment for their child.

The first thing to know is that there are positive options available if you can't afford the cost of treatment. Options include Medicaid and several amazing charity programs.

MEDICAID

If you cannot afford treatment for your child, some state's Medicaid programs will pay for the entire cost of orthodontic treatment for children under the age of nineteen. You must first qualify based on your income and apply for Medicaid in your state of residence. Most states with Medicaid programs that pay for child's orthodontic treatment will have the orthodontist submit records for your child, which include photos, x-rays, and diagnostic models of your child's teeth. However (and it is a big however), even if you qualify for Medicaid, only children with the most severe, most disfiguring orthodontic problems will qualify for no-cost treatment. If your child's orthodontic problems are not severe and they do not qualify, then you may usually appeal the decision with the state. Most appeals, however, are unsuccessful. Most people who qualify for Medicaid are told that their child's case does not qualify for coverage, that their case is not severe enough.[36] These people then go home heartbroken because they really cannot afford to pay for their child's braces. They

---

36   G. Minick et al., "Comparison of Orthodontic Medicaid Funding in the United States 2006 to 2015," Public Health 22 (August 2017), https://doi.org/10.3389/fpubh.2017.00221

end up doing nothing, which is tragic because they don't know that other options exist. Surprisingly, there are great options out there.

It is possible for patients who have some funds and qualify for Medicaid to visit an orthodontic practice that takes Medicaid and charges the Medicaid rate. The potential problem with this is that most Medicaid orthodontic practices see a lot of patients, upward of 150 patients a day. These practices can't run like a private practice does, and they often end up charging you the same amount that Medicaid would have reimbursed them for the case. Many of these offices do not run as efficiently as a private practice and they end up taking a lot longer to finish your treatment than a private office would. For instance, in my state (Illinois), you will be charged upward of $250 every time for an adjustment after the eleventh adjustment visit. Most orthodontic cases go over this amount of adjustments. The number of visits, on average, that are needed in an orthodontic office is fifteen to seventeen adjustments. So, you end up paying just as much for braces as you would have if you had gone to a private provider with a much nicer office, a much more efficient system, and a more-qualified staff. In the end, it would be potentially less expensive and much better quality for those people to go to a private orthodontic provider anyway.

So, if you qualify for Medicaid, but your child's case does not meet the criteria for full coverage *and* you don't want your child to be one of hundreds of patients a day at a Medicaid-reimbursable orthodontic practice (that may cost more), please do not give up. Keep reading. There are great programs available for people like you. We will talk about these programs in the next section.

CHARITY PROGRAMS

There are amazing programs available to help lower-income families pay for orthodontic treatment. Some of them include Smile for a Lifetime, AAO Donated Orthodontic Services, and Smiles Change Lives. These programs are income based, but they usually have less-stringent requirements with regard to the orthodontic problems that will qualify for reduced or no-cost treatment. After all, how are people in this situation ever supposed to become productive members of society so that they can pay for braces if they never have the confidence to raise their hand in class, ask out a date for prom, or go on a job interview?

Many orthodontic practices (including mine) participate in these programs because we *really do* want to make a difference in people's lives. Many orthodontists believe that it is unthinkable that someone will have to endure a lifetime of ridicule because they can't afford braces.

I have treated a lot of patients through the Smiles Change Lives program. Every single one of the parents of patients who I have treated in my office who was part of one of these programs has said to me, "Thank God, we found this, thank God you do this because we couldn't afford to do it and our child's case didn't qualify [for no cost Medicaid coverage]."

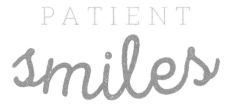

We knew our daughter needed braces, but we really couldn't afford them, and her case was just not severe enough to qualify for full Medicaid coverage. My wife is an avid reader, loves the library, and checks out books on a variety of topics. One day she checked out a book about ways to save money (a

topic of frequent discussion in our home). In this book was a reference to the program Smiles Change Lives. We were pretty excited about this and hopeful that our daughter would qualify for the program. We took pictures of her teeth, our twelve-year-old daughter wrote an essay about why she wanted/needed braces, we completed the application, including a copy of our most recent tax returns, and mailed everything in to the program. It was a pretty easy and smooth process. A few weeks later, we got an e-mail saying that we were approved! We found out Dr. Verbic participates in this program and chose his practice for our daughter's treatment.

Dr. Verbic is phenomenal. Everyone in his practice is really nice and friendly and our daughter is very happy. We really appreciate this program and Dr. Verbic's, and his team's, participation in this program. It is not much, but we try to show how appreciative we are by bringing pastries to the staff. When you are on the lower end of the income spectrum, you aren't always aware of the private programs that are out there and available. In order to help spread the word about Smiles Change Lives, I shared the information with an organization in our community that offers and advertises different types of programs to benefit lower-income people. We want other families to benefit from this amazing program that really does change lives. —**BINYOMIN A.**

A key personal mission of mine is to educate more people about these nonprofit programs that depend on public service announcements for marketing.

Below are the websites for these amazing programs. You will be able to find out all about the particular program, how it works, if you qualify and steps for applying.

- http://www.s4l.org

- https://www.aaoinfo.org/donated-orthodontic-services

- https://www.smileschangelives.org/

SHARING MY HEART

I have a passion for changing lives … one smile at a time.

Although I attended school for seven years after college to become an orthodontist, I realize that having practiced each day for a number of years makes my work less difficult. I know orthodontists' circumstances are all different, but I don't feel it is too difficult to give back, at least a little. The braces and wires don't cost very much and we are already at the office anyway.

I will treat anyone who comes into my practice who needs braces and truly can't afford it. I love working with programs like the ones discussed above. In fact, I find patients treated under these programs to be even more grateful than patients who pay for their treatment. And this is worth so much more to me than money. We all have a higher purpose in life than making money, and giving a life-changing smile to kids that can't afford it is mine.

I feel so strongly about treating children who can't afford braces because the alternative is that they will grow up not being able to raise their hand in class, interview for their first job with confidence, and not follow their desired career paths or dreams. It's a tragedy that can avoided with just a little bit of our time and our talents.

conclusion

CHOOSING THE BEST ORTHODONTIST FOR YOUR CHILD OR YOURSELF

One big question on many people's minds is, "How do I go about finding the right orthodontist for me or for my children?" This question is so important, because at the end of the day, the results are what matters, and your child's smile (and your smile) has to last for the rest of your life. Therefore, you want the best-possible results. When choosing an orthodontic practice that is the best fit for yourself or your child, the following information will help to guide you in your search.

REFERRALS FROM PEOPLE YOU TRUST

I can't think of any better way to find the right orthodontist for you or your child than simply by asking your friends, family members, co-workers, and neighbors where they went for their orthodontic treatment. Where did they go for their children' braces or who did their Invisalign treatment? What was their experience at that practice? Did they like the orthodontist and the people who worked there? Were their children comfortable there? If your children are happy going to the orthodontist instead of dreading every visit, it can make a real difference in your level of satisfaction with the office.

SOCIAL MEDIA ROLE IN CHOOSING A PRACTICE

Another means of evaluating an orthodontic practice today is to explore various social media channels. Does your circle of friends on Facebook, or another social media site, recommend any particular orthodontic practice in your area? What do the online reviews say about the practice in which you are interested? Places to find online reviews include Google and Yelp, but smaller niche review sites that focus on local businesses, such as Angie's List, or on healthcare providers, such as Healthgrades, are additional options. Review sites are certainly less reliable than asking people close to you where they go for their orthodontic treatment, but they can provide an additional means to evaluate a practice.

CREDENTIALS, EDUCATION, AND QUALIFICATIONS OF THE ORTHODONTIST

In addition to who you should ask for a referral or reading online reviews, it is really important to do your research on the orthodontic practice. There are some important things you should look out for when choosing an orthodontist. First and foremost, you want to make sure that the person treating you or your children is a licensed orthodontic specialist. This may seem obvious, but there are some general dentists that push the boundaries of the laws in their state through unscrupulous advertising to make it look like they are specialists.

Legally, dentists are able to provide orthodontic treatment, but this does not mean it is the best choice to have you or your child's treatment performed by a dentist. At this point you may ask yourself, "What's the difference? My dentist says he can treat me and I've been going to him or her for years and trust him or her." The difference is that orthodontists have gone to the same four years of dental school as dentists have, but they have also gone to a residency program for three years after dental school to learn to be orthodontic specialists. This is akin to cardiologists or neurosurgeons going to residency after medical school to specialize in heart surgery or brain surgery, respectively. Ask yourself this question, "Would I want my family doctor performing my heart surgery or my brain surgery?" Orthodontic treatment is no different.

Beyond the additional schooling they receive, orthodontists typically have treated vastly more patients than even the most experienced general dentist. This is because all orthodontists do is treat orthodontic patients. General dentists can do orthodontics, but the overwhelming majority of their days are filled with procedures such as cleanings and exams, and restorative procedures such as fillings, crowns, and dentures. Dentists may treat an orthodontic patient now and then, but they rarely treat enough patients to become as proficient as an orthodontist. Some dentists may feel that they are proficient, but in my experience, few really are, due to the limited number of patients they treat and most of the time it is a case of not knowing what they don't know.

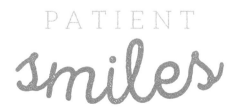

Our oldest daughter had *Invisalign treatment with our family dentist who also practiced orthodontia. Her*

orthodontic case was not very complicated and her teeth were not that crooked or crowded. The Invisalign worked fine for her. However, Madeline, our middle daughter, was not a candidate for Invisalign and her case seemed more complicated. Our family dentist reassured us that, yes, her case was more complicated, but that he could work on her teeth, no problem. Well, he worked on her teeth for over a year with absolutely no progress. I was very fed up and concerned so I asked a trusted friend for a recommendation for a top-quality orthodontist. My friend recommended Dr. Verbic.

We went to see Dr. Verbic and, as politely as he could, he told us he was not sure what our dentist had been doing. He said that the current treatment would never correct our daughter's teeth. That, in fact, a tooth was rotated 180 degrees in the wrong direction! My daughter looked at me and blurted, "See, I told you he was moving my tooth in the wrong direction!" Our daughter's orthodontic treatment took another twenty months, but at least things were moving in the right direction from that point on. —**LINDA G.**

When asked, most orthodontists will tell you they get several transfer patients every month who are unhappy with their orthodontic treatment at their family dentist. This isn't to say there are not some dentists out there who are very good at orthodontics, but it is usually a safer bet to have your and your child's orthodontic treatment performed by an orthodontist.

The best way to tell for sure if an orthodontist is an orthodontist, and not a general dentist, is to look up their license with your state's Department of Professional Regulation. Orthodontists will have a specialty license in orthodontics, whereas a general dentist will not. Another way to make sure is to look up the doctor on the American Association of Orthodontists (AAO) website. Only state-licensed orthodontists are able to belong to the AAO. But be careful. There are many look-alike organizations out there with similar names (e.g., the American Orthodontic Society) that have general dentists and pediatric dentists as members, instead of licensed orthodontists. The official website of the AAO is as follows: www.aaoinfo.org

HOW THE ORTHODONTIC OFFICE IS RUN

In addition to checking and verifying education level and credentials, it is also important to look for an orthodontic practice that has convenient office hours. If you are like most people today, you are very busy. Even the most efficient orthodontic treatment in this day and age requires ten to fifteen visits to the office for adjustments to braces, or five to ten visits for treatment with Invisalign. If evening appointments or weekend appointments work better for you, you should ask if they are available. Some offices will even have early-morning appointments available so that you can still drop the children off at school and make it to work on time. If you miss appointments because a particular practice's hours are not convenient for you, it can extend the length of treatment and cause you to have many more adjustment and repair appointments than are necessary.

In recent years, it has become a popular arrangement for orthodontists to work a couple of days per month in a general dentist's office. This may work well for the dentist and the orthodontist, but does it work well for you to have such limited office hours? What if your child breaks a brace off of their teeth eating something hard or chewing gum? On average, this tends to happens several times throughout treatment. What if something comes up and you can't make it to your appointment? Are you okay with not being able to reschedule for another month and essentially having your treatment progress suspended? I find that most people would like to be seen as soon as possible so that their treatment will finish on time.

THE IMPORTANCE OF GETTING A SECOND OPINION

Visit several of your top picks. Some parents and patients suggest seeking a second opinion in your search for the right orthodontist. And to tell you the truth, I agree. Sometimes, patients will not tell me that they have already seen another orthodontist or they are going for a second opinion after they have seen me. I think they fear that I might be offended. I am never offended. I know that choosing the right orthodontist is a huge decision. Costing several thousand dollars, orthodontic treatment is one of the top expenses in life, right behind buying a car, attending college, or getting married. More importantly, a person's smile, no matter how you or I feel about it, can make an enormous difference in the relationships and opportunities that come their way for the rest of their life. I think getting more than one opinion is a good idea because people should be very comfortable with the orthodontist who is treating them and with their expectations for treatment.

In many instances, quality orthodontists' recommendations are similar, but there can be big differences. Is headgear needed? Are extractions needed? Is surgery needed? Am I candidate for Invisalign? These are questions not all orthodontists agree upon in every patient. Regardless of their recommendations, however, an orthodontist should take the time to thoroughly explain his or her reasoning.

I think it is also fair game to ask the orthodontist for before and after photos of a patient who had similar problems and concerns to yours or your child's prior to having treatment. If your child has a large overbite, ask to see the before and after photos of several children who also had large overbites. If your child has missing teeth, ask to see the photos of children who had the same teeth missing prior to orthodontic treatment. From my perspective, an informed patient who has asked for referrals, done the research, and evaluated another practice and has chosen our practice will have confidence in my office and my recommendations. This patient or parent is more likely to be happy and committed to the treatment program and is more likely to talk highly of my practice and refer friends and family.

QUALITY AND VALUE VERSUS COST

Comparing quality and value to costs is essential in choosing a practice for yourself or your child.

Let's discuss quality first. Higher-cost offices may seem like a bad deal to many people at first. People may think, "This other practice is less expensive and all orthodontics have the same training, so I will spend less for a similar product." This is very often not the case at all. People choose lower-cost practices and then many of them have to seek a second opinion after the less-expensive office fouls things up at the first examination, or even after a year or two of treatment. I am not saying that all lower-cost practices are lower quality, but if a practice wants to attract top talent to work in their office, they need to pay higher salaries, and higher salaries mean that the cost to patients is a bit higher.

Quality aside, value is also a big consideration. Patients at lower-cost practices are often charged for incidentals, so much so that sometimes the less-expensive practice ends up costing more in the end. In addition, lower-cost practices often allow no time for asking questions, and waiting times are often quite long. If you have more time than money, perhaps this is acceptable; it is an individual thing for people.

VALUES OF THE ORTHODONTIC PRACTICE

A final thing to keep in mind when evaluating high-quality orthodontic practices is to ask the staff if their practice participates in programs to help underprivileged kids get orthodontic treatment. An orthodontic practice that gives back to the community shows strong moral and community values.

> *I've had so much fun writing a book about the thing I love to do most in this world: creating beautiful smiles. I hope I answered some of your questions. Maybe I raised some new questions? Maybe the stories from some of my patients, co-workers, friends, family members, and myself have inspired you or changed the way you think about orthodontics. Maybe these words have convinced you to go for an orthodontic consult after years of thinking about it or putting it off until you had more time or more money. Maybe these words have convinced you to take your child in for an orthodontic consult earlier than you thought you would to get an opinion on the need for early treatment. Perhaps these words have even encouraged you to donate to programs that help needy families afford treatment for their children. I hope so; I really do. I love to talk about orthodontics and teeth almost as much as I like to work on them, so if you have more questions or a story of your own you would like to share, check out my website and leave me a message.*
>
> **—DR. VERBIC**

PALATINEBRACES.COM

Printed in the USA
CPSIA information can be obtained
at www.ICGtesting.com
JSHW072029140824
68134JS00045B/3844